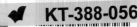

Recent Advances in

Obstetrics & Gynaecology 25

Recent Advances in

Obstetrics & Gynaecology
25

William Ledger MA DPhil FRCOG FRANZCOG CREI
Professor of Obstetrics and Gynaecology
Royal Hospital for Women
Randwick, Australia

Justin Clark MD MRCOG
Department of Obstetrics and Gynaecology
Birmingham Women's Hospital
Birmingham, UK

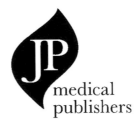

JP
medical
publishers

London • Philadelphia • Panama City • New Delhi

© 2014 JP Medical Ltd.
Published by JP Medical Ltd,
83 Victoria Street, London, SW1H 0HW, UK
Tel: +44 (0)20 3170 8910   Fax: +44 (0)20 3008 6180
Email: info@jpmedpub.com   Web: www.jpmedpub.com

ISBN: 978-1-907816-80-2

British Library Cataloguing in Publication Data
A catalogue record for this book is available from the British Library

Library of Congress Cataloging in Publication Data
A catalog record for this book is available from the Library of Congress

JP Medical Ltd is a subsidiary of Jaypee Brothers Medical Publishers (P) Ltd, New Delhi, India

Commissioning Editor: Steffan Clements
Editorial Assistant: Sophie Woolven
Design: Designers Collective Ltd

Copy edited, typeset, indexed, printed and bound in India.

Preface

In keeping with the tradition of the *Recent Advances* series, we have aimed to provide a collection of reviews of significant areas in which there have been new developments or changes in practice in our speciality. Whilst it is impossible to cover the entire breadth of this ever-changing speciality, subject diversity has been one of our criteria when selecting chapters to include in *Recent Advances in Obstetrics & Gynaecology 25*.

To exemplify this diversity, the content highlights areas such as fetal medicine, which is increasingly utilising non-invasive techniques for prenatal diagnosis. There are chapters on the mechanisms behind parturition, the challenge of stillbirth and optimisation of the management of high risk mothers, such as those with cardiac disease, all of which remain relevant in day-to-day obstetric practice. Packages of care designed to enhance recovery after caesarean section and gynaecological surgery have recently been proposed and are covered here. Best practice in the management of common conditions in general gynaecology and early pregnancy are also explored, along with new thinking about the regulation of reproduction and the treatment of infertile couples. In oncology, the role of genetics and infection in gynaecological cancer are reviewed.

Systematic reviews provide evidence-based summaries to answer focussed clinical questions. However, the wider overview of an area of practice – as provided by the high quality, contemporary, narrative reviews in this volume – is invaluable to busy clinicians, especially those preparing for examinations. We hope you find the content of this volume of *Recent Advances in Obstetrics & Gynaecology* edifying and enjoyable.

William Ledger
Justin Clark
May 2014

Contents

Chapter 1

The role of laparoscopy and cystoscopy in the diagnosis and management of chronic pelvic and bladder pain

Seema A Tirlapur, Khalid S Khan, Elizabeth Ball

BACKGROUND

Chronic pelvic pain (CPP) in women has prevalence rates comparable to that of lower back pain and asthma, causing a huge impact on the quality of life of the individual patient and a large burden on the economy [1]. In this chapter, we explore the role of laparoscopy as a diagnostic and therapeutic tool in the management of CPP. We investigate bladder pain syndrome (BPS) as a manifestation of CPP and the role cystoscopy plays in its diagnosis and treatment. We also explore the causes of CPP and evaluate the most effective methods of diagnosis.

WHAT IS CHRONIC PELVIC PAIN?

Chronic pelvic pain is an intermittent or constant pain in the lower abdomen for at least 6 months, not associated with pregnancy and not occurring exclusively with menstruation or sexual intercourse [2]. The International Association for the Study of Pain and the European Association of Urology revised definition of CPP includes both men and women, with pain perceived in structures related to the pelvis, acknowledging its negative impact on cognition, behaviour, sexual and emotional well-being and noting the possible association with urinary, bowel, sexual, pelvic floor or gynaecological dysfunction [3, 4].

There is difficulty in delineating causes behind CPP as there are many possible causes for the pain and several pathologies may co-exist, making a single diagnosis sometimes impossible. A recent systematic review estimated the prevalence of CPP to range between

Seema A Tirlapur MBChB, Women's Health Research Unit, Queen Mary, University of London, London, UK.
Email: s.a.tirlapur@qmul.ac.uk (for correspondence)

Khalid S Khan MRCOG MMed MSc, Women's Health Research Unit, Queen Mary, University of London, UK.

Elizabeth Ball MD PhD MRCOG, Barts Health NHS Trust, The Royal London Hospital, London, UK.

8–81% worldwide [5]. The range of causes for CPP is extensive and the methods of diagnosis for each vary in terms of diagnostic accuracy and patient acceptability. The causes of CPP may be classified as gynaecological versus non-gynaecological or structural and non-structural. Gynaecological causes include endometriosis, adenomyosis, ovarian cysts, uterine fibroids, pelvic congestion syndrome, chronic pelvic inflammatory disease (PID) and adhesions, which may be gynaecological, secondary to endometriosis or PID or non-gynaecological after previous surgery or infection. Non-gynaecological causes include irritable bowel syndrome and BPS as well as musculoskeletal, neuropathic and psychological conditions.

THE ROLE OF LAPAROSCOPY

More than 250,000 laparoscopies are performed annually in the United Kingdom. Diagnostic laparoscopy has been regarded as the 'gold standard' investigation for CPP, after a careful preoperative work-up, which involves a thorough history, physical examination and imaging in the form of pelvic ultrasound or pelvic magnetic resonance imaging, if necessary [2]. However, depending on the preceding work-up, up to 40% of diagnostic laparoscopies fail to show any pathological cause for the patient's pain [6].

Table 1.1 shows the gynaecological causes of CPP and the accuracy of laparoscopy as a diagnostic tool. Laparoscopy can successfully diagnose adhesions and several types of endometriosis [6, 7], but its accuracy in diagnosing other pathologies associated with CPP is unproven. Nevertheless, diagnostic laparoscopy remains a popular test in the work-up of CPP and this may reflect its additional benefits. These include assessment of fertility

Table 1.1 Gynaecological causes of chronic pelvic pain and the accuracy of laparoscopy as a diagnostic tool		
Target condition	Diagnostic criteria	Role of laparoscopy
Adenomyosis	Presence of islands of ectopic endometrial tissue within the myometrium confirmed histologically	Uncertain value – appearance bulky 'boggy' uterus
Adhesions	Visual inspection during laparoscopy, or by absence of movement between adjacent organs	Gold standard – visual inspection
Endometriosis	Visual inspection during laparoscopy, noting appearance, size and depth of endometrial implants	Gold standard – negative laparoscopy can exclude disease but positive findings cannot accurately confirm disease [13]
Fibroids	Size and location noted during pelvic ultrasound	Uncertain – visual inspection of size and location of subserosal fibroids
Ovarian cysts	Pelvic ultrasound or magnetic resonance imaging to define size, location and nature of cyst, confirmed histologically	Uncertain value – visual inspection of size and location of cyst
Pelvic congestion syndrome	Definitive diagnosis on catheter-directed venography, showing uterine venous engorgement and ovarian complex congestion [29]	Uncertain value – appearance of pelvic varicosities
Pelvic inflammatory disease	Visual inspection during laparoscopy or histology from fimbrial biopsy [30]	Uncertain value – may identify salpingitis, adhesions and Fitz-Hugh-Curtis syndrome

by examining tubal patency, and evaluating the severity of disease to plan appropriate treatment, e.g. identifying the presence of severe endometriosis necessitating management in an experienced endometriosis centre.

Laparoscopy requires insertion of instruments into the peritoneal cavity and is not without risk, highlighted by the fact that up to 57% of gynaecologists have reported major bowel and vascular injures, regardless of the entry technique used [8]. Whilst laparoscopy is more invasive than other testing modalities in CPP, the technique allows surgical treatments to be effected enhanced by advances in instrumentation. Thus, in an attempt to avoid multiple operations and their associated surgical and anaesthetic risks, 'see and treat' therapeutic laparoscopies are considered preferable [9]. To successfully achieve such an efficient approach to managing CPP requires good prior diagnostic work up. For example, in addition to thorough clinical assessment, a rigorously performed pelvic ultrasound scan may be useful. Feature suggestive of endometriosis or adhesions can be detected such as site-specific pain of the uterosacral ligaments, decreased ovarian mobility, presence of endometriomas and hydrosalpinges [10]. The surgeon can then more effectively plan the site and setting for surgery and ensure that the patient is well informed and that suitably skilled staff and surgical instruments are available [9].

Endometriosis

Endometriosis often affects areas of the pelvis, such as the uterosacral ligaments, pouch of Douglas and rectovaginal septum, which are difficult to assess clinically [11]. Laparoscopy can improve diagnostic accuracy but has limitations. One observational study noted that 42% of general gynaecologists failed to recognise rectovaginal endometriosis on visual inspection at primary laparoscopy [12]. A systematic review of the accuracy of laparoscopic visual inspection in the diagnosis of peritoneal endometriosis showed that a negative laparoscopy could accurately exclude endometriosis, whilst a positive laparoscopy needed to be followed by histological confirmation [13]. The technique of diagnostic laparoscopy is important such that a careful, systematic inspection of the abdomen and pelvis is undertaken and importantly adequate anteversion and anteflexion of the uterus is achieved to allow for thorough inspection of the pouch of Douglas. Despite these limitations, most gynaecologists view visual inspection at laparoscopy as the 'gold standard' method of diagnosing superficial endometriosis.

Superficial peritoneal endometriosis can be treated by cautery or excision. There is much debate over the optimal method of treating superficial endometriosis and often depends on the surgeons preference. Whilst excision is effective and enables a histological biopsy to be obtained for disease confirmation, it requires dissection skills and knowledge of underlying structures to avoid trauma. Excision also allows visualisation of possible invasion below diseased areas, especially of uterosacral ligament endometriosis. In contrast, ablative treatments may be inadequate due to the risk of thermal injury to nearby structures. A small randomised controlled trial (RCT) of 24 patients, compared ablation using monopolar diathermy versus excision using monopolar diathermy scissors in patients with mild endometriosis (stage 1 or 2 revised American Fertility Score). Both methods of treatment produced symptomatic relief with no difference between the treatments with regard to 6-month symptom questionnaire scores [14]. A large randomised trial is needed to compare diathermy versus excision to obtain more reliable results.

Adhesions

Adhesions may be caused by endometriosis, exposure to infection or previous surgery and can cause pain by organ distension or stretching [2]. They can range from fine filmy adhesions to dense, vascular ones. The symptomatic benefits of laparoscopic adhesiolysis are uncertain. Whilst there is no clear evidence to support adhesiolysis in women with CPP, an RCT of 100 patients treated with adhesiolysis compared to no treatment during diagnostic laparoscopy for chronic abdominal pain, showed both groups reported substantial pain relief with no difference between the groups 1 year after surgery [15]. Similar results were noted in a small observational study, with 45% of patients reporting on-going symptomatic relief 2 years after laparoscopic adhesiolysis [16]. From these results, it can be argued that there may be a psychologically beneficial effect to surgery and the perceived improvement in pain [17].

Adenomyosis

Adenomyosis is a common benign gynaecological condition, often reported on imaging or identified during laparoscopy. It is defined by the presence of islands of ectopic endometrial tissue within the myometrium, causing smooth muscle hypertrophy [18A]. It can be associated with endometriosis and endometrial hyperplasia and is known to cause heavy menstrual bleeding and dysmenorrhoea. On laparoscopy, the clinician may observe the classical appearance of a bulky 'boggy' uterus, although the accuracy of laparoscopic diagnosis is unproven and final diagnosis rests upon histological confirmation, usually after hysterectomy. Imaging in the form of pelvic ultrasound or magnetic resonance imaging (MRI) may identify the condition with good accuracy (72% sensitivity for transvaginal ultrasound and 77% for MRI, compared against histology), allowing medical treatment to be initiated without the need for surgery [18B].

UNCERTAINTIES OF LAPAROSCOPY

A diagnostic laparoscopy can be a useful tool for evaluating the causes of CPP, but 40% of laparoscopies may show no pathology. Clinicians should therefore carefully weigh up the perceived surgical benefits of laparoscopy against the risks of surgery. Patients need to be informed about the limitations of this investigation and the implications of a 'negative' laparoscopy. CPP has many non-gynaecological and non-structural causes, which may not be identified by laparoscopy, e.g. functional and psychosomatic conditions which may benefit from alternative complementary therapies. The term chronic pelvic pain syndrome (CPPS) has been introduced by the International Association for the Study of Pain to describe the occurrence of CPP where pain may be focused around a single organ or multiple pelvic organs, and where there is no proven infection or other obvious local pathology to account for the pain [4]. Whilst a laparoscopy may not always be able to identify any cause of pain, sometimes this can have a beneficial, reassuring effect on the patient [19].

WHAT IS BLADDER PAIN SYNDROME?

Patients suffering from BPS may present with CPP. BPS is the condition formerly known as interstitial cystitis and painful bladder syndrome. It is defined as CPP, pressure or discomfort related to the bladder along with at least one other urinary symptom, such as urgency or frequency, in the absence of any other pathology [20]. The prevalence of BPS is estimated to be between 2 and 306 per 100,000 of the population, with lower prevalence in the Japanese population compared to European and American patients [21]. There is variation in the method of diagnosing BPS because patients may present with a wide spectrum of pain and urinary symptoms, which makes accurate prevalence rates difficult to record.

In 2008, The International Society for the Study of BPS suggested that BPS may be classified according to the findings at cystoscopy, hydrodistension and bladder biopsies with a normal cystoscopy equating to BPS grade 1, glomerulations (pin point sized areas of bleeding) equating to grade 2 and Hunner's lesions (distinctive areas of inflammation) were grade 3 with sub-classification a, b, or c depending on biopsy results [20]. **Table 1.2** shows the classification of BPS according to cystoscopy and biopsy findings. In some previous guidelines, BPS has traditionally been defined and diagnosed through cystoscopy findings alone [21]. In 2011, the American Association of Urology (AUA) published guidelines on the diagnosis and management of BPS, which recommend that initial assessments should include a careful history, physical examination and laboratory tests to exclude infection. An important recommendation is that cystoscopy may be used as an aid in complex cases but it is not necessary to make a diagnosis or commence treatment [22]. Conservative first-line treatments, such as stress and pain management, patient education and and lifestyle modifications such as change in diet, avoidance of caffeine and limiting evening fluid intake, should be initiated without delays.

THE ROLE OF CYSTOSCOPY

Cystoscopy is often thought of as the investigation of choice to diagnose BPS. It can differentiate between BPS with normal bladder mucosal appearance from grade 2 and 3 disease with the presence of petechial bleeds, glomerulations and Hunner's lesions/ulcers [23]. The presence of Hunner's ulcers may lead the clinician to offer alternative treatments such as fulguration at an early stage, rather than persevering with conservative treatments. Hydrodistension during cystoscopy can allow visualisation of petechial haemorrhages. It can also provoke petechial bleeds that are thought to be pathognomonic.

Table 1.2 Classification of bladder pain syndrome according to cystoscopy and biopsy findings [20]				
	Cystoscopy with hydrodistension			
	Not done	Normal	Glomerulations [b]	Hunner's lesions [c]
Biopsy:				
Not done	XX	1X	2X	3X
Normal	XA	1A	2A	3A
Inconclusive	XB	1B	2B	3B
Positive [a]	XC	1C	2C	3C

[a] Histology showing inflammatory infiltrates and/or detrusor mastocytosis and/or granulation tissue and/or intrafasicular fibrosis.
[b] Glomerulations: grade 2 (several areas of submucosal bleeding) and grade 3 (diffuse bleeding of bladder mucosa).
[c] With or without glomerulations.

Cystoscopy with hydrodistension has a therapeutic effect. The hydropressure is believed to degenerate afferent nerves, leading to reduced bladder pain and increased bladder capacity [21]. If brief hydrodistension is performed, using 80–100 cm of water for 2–10 minutes, studies have shown variable symptomatic improvement but the effects decreased after 6 months post treatment [24]. Prolonged periods of hydrodistension are not recommended due to the adverse effect of bladder rupture [22].

THE UNCERTAINTIES OF CYSTOSCOPY

Cystoscopy and bladder biopsies have traditionally been used as the 'gold standard' to diagnose and classify BPS [20]. However, some studies show poor correlation between cystoscopy findings and diagnosis, because glomerulations may be seen in asymptomatic patients and bladder biopsies may not confirm disease in the presence of glomerulations [21, 25]. This has resulted in uncertainties in the diagnosis and management of the BPS. Some guidance ranks diagnosis by cystoscopy ahead of bladder biopsy when recommending evidence-based treatments [23]. Guidance from the AUA recognises the limitations of cystoscopy and bladder biopsy. It supports a clinical diagnosis, based upon symptoms and signs derived from the patient history and examination, on which to recommend treatment [22].

CONCLUSION

There are many causes for CPP. Several risk factors, such as a history of drug, alcohol and sexual abuse, PID, anxiety and depression have been associated with CPP [26]. In order to fully investigate a patient and possibly diagnose the cause of pain, invasive procedures like a laparoscopy and cystoscopy may be useful and can have therapeutic effects. The degree of sensitivity of each test varies with the target condition, and these procedures may not yield a cause of pain, which may reassure some patients but equally may cause distress if no obvious cause of pain can be identified [19]. Prior to surgery, a careful work-up of the patient with thorough history, examination and imaging is essential to correctly plan management. When a laparoscopy is performed, a 'see and treat' therapeutic laparoscopy is recommended rather than a purely diagnostic procedure, provided the surgeon is suitably trained and equipped.

CPP and BPS affect large numbers of people across the world, often with unknown etiology and overlapping symptoms and possibly co-existing disease pathology, which makes the management of such patients difficult [27, 28]. Both conditions may have non-specific symptoms with pain as the main complaint. In light of these considerations, it may be prudent to perform both laparoscopy and cystoscopy in cases of persistent CPP.

Key points for clinical practice

- CPP can be due to structural or non-structural causes.
- CPP may be due to multiple co-existing pathologies.
- Laparoscopy is useful in the diagnosis of endometriosis and adhesions and in the assessment of the severity of disease.
- The need for laparoscopy should be based upon clinical information obtained from the patient history and examination, as well as the findings from preceding radiological imaging.
- Cystoscopy can be used as a therapeutic treatment for BPS.
- Laparoscopy and cystoscopy are useful investigations to rule out gynaecological and bladder pathology and so should be routinely considered in persistent CPP.

REFERENCES

1. Zondervan KT, Yudkin PL, Vessey MP, et al. Prevalence and incidence of chronic pelvic pain in primary care: evidence from a national general practice database. Br J Obstet Gynaecol. 1999; 106:1149–1155.
2. Royal College of Obstetricians and Gynaecologists. Initial management of chronic pelvic pain 2012; 27:2712–2719.
3. Engeler D, Baranowski AP, Elneil S, et al. Guidelines on Chronic Pelvic Pain. Arnhem: European Association of Urology 2012.
4. Baranowski A, Abrams P, Berger R, et al. Classification of Chronic Pain, 2nd edn. Washington: International Association for the Study of Pain, 2011.
5. Latthe P, Latthe M, Say L, et al. WHO systematic review of prevalence of chronic pelvic pain: a neglected reproductive health morbidity. BMC Public Health 2006; 6:177.
6. Howard FM. The role of laparoscopy in chronic pelvic pain: promise and pitfalls. Obstet Gynecol Surv. 1993; 48:357–387.
7. Hebbar S, Chawla C. Role of laparoscopy in evaluation of chronic pelvic pain. J Minim Access Surg. 2005; 1:116–120.
8. Ahmad G, O'Flynn H, Duffy JM, et al. Laparoscopic entry techniques. Cochrane Database Syst Rev. 2012; 2:CD006583.
9. Ball E, Koh C, Janik G, et al. Gynaecological laparoscopy: 'see and treat' should be the gold standard. Curr Opin Obstet Gynecol 2008; 20:325–330.
10. Okaro E, Condous G, Khalid A, et al. The use of ultrasound-based 'soft markers' for the prediction of pelvic pathology in women with chronic pelvic pain – can we reduce the need for laparoscopy? BJOG 2006; 113:251–256.
11. Byrne H, Ball E, Davis C. The role of magnetic resonance imaging in minimal access surgery. Curr Opin Obstet Gynecol. 2006; 18:369–373
12. Griffiths AN, Koutsouridou RN, Penketh RJ. Rectovaginal endometriosis – a frequently missed diagnosis. J Obstet Gynaecol 2007; 27:605–607.
13. Wykes CB, Clark TJ, Khan KS. Accuracy of laparoscopy in the diagnosis of endometriosis: a systematic quantitative review. BJOG 2004; 111:1204–1212.
14. Wright J, Lotfallah H, Jones K, et al. A randomized trial of excision versus ablation for mild endometriosis. Fertil Steril 2005; 83:1830–1836.
15. Swank DJ, Swank-Bordewijk SC, Hop WC, et al. Laparoscopic adhesiolysis in patients with chronic abdominal pain: a blinded randomised controlled multi-centre trial. Lancet 2003; 361:1247–1251.
16. Dunker MS, Bemelman WA, Vijn A, et al. Long-term outcomes and quality of life after laparoscopic adhesiolysis for chronic abdominal pain. J Am Assoc Gynecol Laparosc 2004; 11:36–41.
17. Elcombe S, Gath D, Day A. The psychological effects of laparoscopy on women with chronic pelvic pain. Psychol Med 1997; 27:1041–1050.
18A.Levy G, Dehaene A, Laurent N, et al. An update on adenomyosis. Diagn Interv Imaging 2013; 94:3–25.

18B. Champaneria R, Abedin P, Daniels J, et al. Ultrasound scan and magnetic resonance imaging for the diagnosis of adenomyosis: systematic review comparing test accuracy. Acta Obstet Gynecol Scand 2010;89:1374-84.

19. Yasmin H, Bombieri L, Hollingworth J. What happens to women with chronic pelvic pain after a negative [normal] laparoscopy? J Obstet Gynaecol 2005; 25:283–285.

20. van de Merwe JP, Nordling J, Bouchelouche P, et al. Diagnostic criteria, classification, and nomenclature for painful bladder syndrome/interstitial cystitis: an ESSIC proposal. Eur Urol 2008; 53:60–67.

21. Homma Y, Ueda T, Ito T, et al. Japanese guideline for diagnosis and treatment of interstitial cystitis. Int J Urol 2009; 16:4–16.

22. Hanno PM, Burks DA, Clemens JQ, et al. AUA guideline for the diagnosis and treatment of interstitial cystitis/bladder pain syndrome. J Urol 2011; 185:2162–2170.

23. Offiah I, McMahon SB, O'Reilly BA. Interstitial cystitis/bladder pain syndrome: diagnosis and management. Int Urogynecol J. 2013; 24:1243–1256.

24. Rigaud J, Delavierre D, Sibert L, et al. Hydrodistension in the therapeutic management of painful bladder syndrome. Prog Urol 2010; 20:1054–1059.

25. Cheng C, Rosamilia A, Healey M. Diagnosis of interstitial cystitis/bladder pain syndrome in women with chronic pelvic pain: a prospective observational study. Int Urogynecol J 2012; 23:1361–1366.

26. Latthe P, Mignini L, Gray R, et al. Factors predisposing women to chronic pelvic pain: systematic review. BMJ 2006; 332:749–755.

27. Tirlapur SA, Kuhrt K, Chaliha C, et al The 'evil twin syndrome' in chronic pelvic pain: a systematic review of prevalence studies of bladder pain syndrome and endometriosis. Int J Surg 2013; 11:233–237.

28. Butrick CW. Patients with chronic pelvic pain: endometriosis or interstitial cystitis/painful bladder syndrome? JSLS 2007; 11:182–189.

29. Freedman J, Ganeshan A, Crowe PM. Pelvic congestion syndrome: the role of interventional radiology in the treatment of chronic pelvic pain. Postgrad Med J 2010; 86:704–710.

30. Munday PE. Clinical aspects of pelvic inflammatory disease. Hum Reprod 1997; 12:121–126.

Chapter 2

Enhanced recovery in obstetric and gynaecological surgery

Robin Crawford, Nigel Acheson

BACKGROUND

Enhanced recovery (ER) is an evidence based model of care for elective surgery that enables patients to recover more quickly and leave hospital sooner. Every aspect of the pathway from decision to discharge is planned to promote good outcomes and rapid return to normal function. Enhanced recovery was first described in the 1990s by Professor Kehlet [1] in Denmark who introduced a different standard of care in colorectal surgery. Adherence to a standardised, predefined care pathway resulted in reduced the physiological stress of surgery such that patients recovered more quickly, allowing discharge from hospital after 2–3 days and without increased surgical morbidity. At the time this ER package was introduced, the standard length of stay (LoS) in UK hospitals for a colon resection was over 2 weeks.

Application of the principles of ER across a number of surgical specialities has been recognised by the Department of Health (DH) and others as advantageous in that tangible benefits could potentially be delivered to both patients and the wider health service. Quality of care for patients could be improved helping them to recover more quickly after surgery. Furthermore, health service capacity could be enhanced by reducing the number of bed days used for common surgical interventions. In 2009, the enhanced recovery partnership programme, an initiative between the DH, the National Cancer Action Team, the NHS Improvement Agency and the NHS institute commenced. The programme built on the principles of ER expanding the remit to include gynaecology, urology and musculoskeletal surgery.

However, implementation of novel ER care packages is difficult. In many instances, established principles of surgical management, the origins of which can often be traced back more than 60 years, are challenged. Introducing new approaches to patient care and discarding many embedded, traditional practises requires training and support.

Robin Crawford MD FRCOG, Department of Gynaecology, Addenbrookes Hospital, Cambridge University Hospitals NHS Foundation Trust, Cambridge, UK. Email: robin.crawford@addenbrookes.nhs.uk (for correspondence)

Nigel Acheson MD PGCert (Patient Safety and Risk Management) FRCOG, Royal Devon and Exeter NHS Foundation Trust, Taunton, UK.

ENHANCED RECOVERY AND GYNAECOLOGY

Surgical pathways using the elements of enhanced recovery reduce the physical and psychological impact of elective gynaecological surgery on the patient to facilitate a more rapid recovery from surgery and return to normal activity. A consensus view of experts, chosen from teams with experience of delivering a successful ER after surgery programmes across different surgical specialties and across various disciplines [2], suggested that 60% of gynaecological patients would either gain moderate or great benefit from being managed using ER principles.

Hysterectomy is the commonest major operation performed in elective gynaecology. There is significant variation in both the hysterectomy rate and the mode of hysterectomy across England [4]. Understanding the causes of this variation is important to ensure that the most appropriate type of hysterectomy is performed according to the needs of each patient. There are a number of possible explanations for the variation observed. The authors consider that for benign cases, all other factors being equal, that the surgical approach should be vaginal or laparoscopic, with abdominal incisions reserved for cases in which other considerations such as previous surgery, complex pathology or a very large uterus are present. In Finland, an active move to change the route of hysterectomy in benign surgery from the abdominal approach to either laparoscopic or vaginal modes has been successful leading to shorter length of stay. Comparing 2006 to the decade previously, there were 34% fewer hysterectomies performed and the abdominal route changed from 58% to 24% with an increase in laparoscopic and vaginal procedures [5].

Involving the patient at every step of the process from decision to discharge by making them partners in their care is a fundamental part of ER pathways (**Figure 2.1**). Patients who are more informed and involved have an improved experience of their care. The implementation of ER pathways can be associated with improved quality of life following surgery, compared to traditional pathways [6].

PRINCIPLES OF ENHANCED RECOVERY

Preoperative intervention

Primary care

Assessment of a patient's health and fitness for a surgical procedure should be timed to allow optimisation of any problems identified. This process should start in the community prior to referral and continue in preadmission clinics. This can be achieved by the primary care doctor reviewing general health and optimising preexisting long-term conditions and medication at the time of referral. In the benign setting, the general practitioner can advise the patient to reduce or stop smoking, to lose weight if required and to improve fitness. Active interventions such as checking blood pressure and diabetic control or optimising asthma management are important contributory factors to successful ER pathways. In those patients where there is a suspected cancer and surgical intervention deemed urgent, this preparation may be limited to information and advice. However, in approximately 10% of gynaecological cancer patients, major comorbidity is present and this will need to be optimised as far as possible during the hospital preadmission process (personal communication Crawford R, 2014).

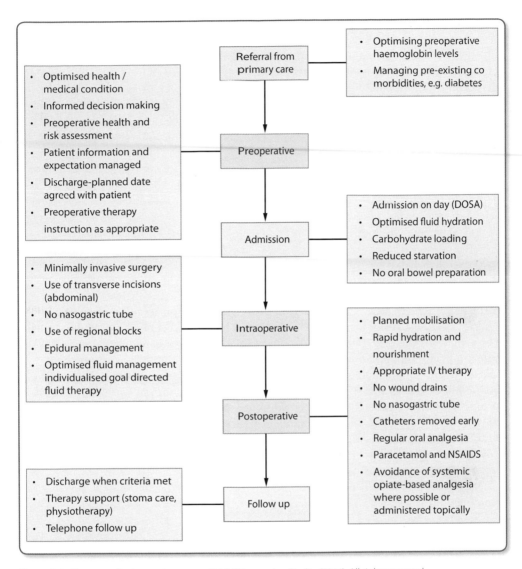

Figure 2.1 Elements of enhanced recovery. © NHS Improving Quality (2014). All rights reserved.

Secondary care

Hospital preadmission assessment is important to address correctable problems and optimise those which cannot be eradicated. In particular appropriate anaesthetic input can be accessed and the correct perioperative location such as the elective use of high dependency or intensive care units. Whilst there is an element of urgency in the pathway for patients with suspected malignancy, the ER process works well to support patients by allowing them to participate in their care at a very stressful time.

Comprehensive verbal and written patient information helps to ensure that patients understand the pathway that they will follow, and crucially the active part that they will play in their care. Furthermore informed decision making following discussion about the options for treatment can lead to greater satisfaction with the outcome of surgery [3]. Procedure specific information and consent can greatly aid the information giving phase of the preadmission process. The use of procedure specific consent forms allow consistent peer reviewed information to be given to patients, and also streamlines consenting on the day of surgery. This information should be up to date and be reviewed regularly. Poor information can confuse the patient and carers and reduce their active participation in the process. The key role of specialist nurses or surgical care practitioners in ER cannot be overstated. Day of surgery admission is now standard in units following the successful introduction of ER and is one simple way to achieve early significant cost savings.

Preoperative planning for the day of discharge is another key element of ER pathways. Information about the expected length of stay for a particular procedure helps ensure that patient, their relatives, carers and community agencies, can provide appropriate support at the time of planned discharge.

Perioperative intervention

Non-surgical intervention

On the day of surgery, dehydration is avoided by reducing the period of starvation to 2 hours for clear fluids prior to anaesthetic. The use of complex carbohydrate drinks, shown to be beneficial in colorectal surgery [7], reduces LoS. Comprising mainly maltodextrins, these drinks are emptied from the stomach within 2 hours and provide a carbohydrate meal to ensure optimal metabolic conditioning. This approach not only reduces thirst and preoperative dehydration, but also leads to a reduction in patient anxiety, a reduced postoperative insulin resistance, reduced postoperative nitrogen and protein losses and improved grip strength [8]. The appropriate preoperative hydration of patients reduces postoperative nausea and vomiting as well as headaches. This leads to more consistent early discharge. Bowel preparation is avoided as it has no benefit [9A]. Avoiding long-acting sedative premedication aids postoperative mobilisation.

Consideration and inclusion where appropriate of preoperative antibiotics and venous thromboembolic prophylaxis is important in evidenced based care bundles.

Surgical and anaesthetic intervention

The use of minimal access techniques is supported [9B,9C]. An abdominal incision, when used, should be as small as possible to allow the safe and appropriate surgery. Routine use of drains and packs should be avoided [10A,10B]. Avoidance of intraoperative hypothermia reduces postoperative complications [10C]. Physiologically-guided, individualised fluid administration known as goal directed fluid therapy (GDFT), allows optimal hydration intraoperatively by assessing stroke volume. This is important for colorectal surgery because it reduces the risk of bowel hypoperfusion, but the role in gynaecological surgery is less clear. A study in a gynaecological oncology centre showed there was a quicker postoperative recovery and an earlier fitness for discharge in women with advanced disease when oesophageal Doppler was used for GDFT [11]. No benefit was seen for early or benign disease.

Reducing variation in anaesthetic protocols may improve patient outcomes and promotes patient safety. Spinal, epidural and regional analgesia regimes do not prolong recovery and reduce opiate requirements [12]. In meta-analyses, adjuvants such as magnesium [13, 14], ketorolac [15], lidocaine [16] ketamine [17] and gabapentin [18] have all been shown to reduce the postoperative pain and opiate consumption.

Some units are evaluating rectus sheath catheters, which use local anaesthetic, as an alternative to epidural analgesia for midline incisions [19]. It is important for the gynaecologist and anaesthetist to produce a workable 'cocktail' that suites their practice. Liaison between gynaecologists and anaesthetists should try and identify successful regimens which could be standardised to reduce variation and risks within gynaecology departments.

Postoperative

Early feeding should be encouraged with a reduction in the volume of routine intravenous fluid infusion [20]. Early mobilisation is realised by reducing systemic opiates, using effective oral analgesia and antiemetic regimes and removing urinary catheters early. Spinal anaesthesia for abdominal hysterectomy is associated with less morphine usage, better patient satisfaction and more rapid return to work but not associated with shorter hospital stay [21,6,22].

Discharge

Discharge criteria for patients on ER pathways are criteria based. Patients should be discharged when they are mobilising, can control their pain by oral analgesia, are able to eat and drink, voiding urine and passing flatus. In our experience, patients treated as day case or short stay (23 hours) hysterectomy following minimal invasive surgical techniques can safely be discharged along ER pathways. Patients who are unable to void urine satisfactorily at their initial 'trial without catheter' can have the catheter replaced and sent home and the indwelling urinary catheter removed at a subsequent outpatient visit a few days later. Patients should be provided with written information on discharge that includes emergency contact information, practical advice to aid recovery and expected length of time until they return to normal function. Typically, there is no increase in readmissions or postoperative work for primary care [23]. Reviewing Hospital Episode Statistics in England since 2010 has not shown an increase in readmissions as the enhanced recovery concept has been introduced. The authors experience with over 3 years of active ER programmes in two gynaecological cancer centres in England has shown that emergency phone lines are seldom used and easy access to the ward and specialist nurses achieve high levels of safety and patient satisfaction.

Those patients who are not fit for discharge should be monitored carefully because this may be an early sign of postoperative complications.

QUALITY AND COST

There is little net investment required for the successful introduction of ER pathways. Enhanced recovery releases beds for either increased activity or savings. Length of stay data is readily available from DH Hospital Episode Statistics (HES) allowing inter-hospital comparison; arguably such data can be taken as a surrogate marker for quality of care as shorter stays suggest fewer complications.

Another marker of quality is patient satisfaction, collected by the inpatient survey, questionnaires or patient diaries. Overall patient feedback supports ER. Locally, readmissions should be investigated and issues addressed. To date there has not been an increase in re-admissions nationally according to available HES data. Reducing variation within departments and across Trusts will help with the quality agenda.

IMPLEMENTATION

Successful implementation of ER involves input from all parts of the healthcare community from primary and social care through to secondary care. In secondary care, engagement of clinical and management teams at high level is required for the sustained introduction of ER.

In England, until the end of March 2013 there was support and information available to trusts planning to implement ER from the national website http://www.improvement.nhs.uk/enhancedrecovery and in the document 'delivering enhanced recovery' published by the enhanced recovery partnership programme. The online resources can still be accessed via NHS IQ, and this site contains contact details for those who require further information.

EVIDENCE

The benefits of ER seem intuitive but high quality evidence to support widespread adoption of ER is scarce. Chase [24] reported a retrospective review of cancer patients with a short LoS and Kalogera [25] reported the benefits of ER across major cancer and benign gynaecological cases compared with historical controls. Complication and readmission rates were comparable to, or better than those seen in the UK [24]. A Cochrane review [26] highlighted that there were no randomised trials in ER. As ER is a relatively new concept for gynaecology, it is not surprising about the absence of randomised trials. The effective key components of ER need to be further elucidated. For example, maintaining the patient's body temperature during and after surgery is associated with less postoperative complications [27]. There are a number of randomised studies into elements of the ER pathway underway; optimal postoperative analgesia is an area of ongoing study.

Informed decision making appears to help women make the appropriate decision with respect to treatment options including surgery [3]. Concerns about the shorter LoS reducing patient access to information and education appear to be unfounded. Enhanced recovery programmes seem to give better patient satisfaction together with the reduced LoS [28].

FUTURE DEVELOPMENTS

The concept of ER is applicable to all gynaecology departments and ER pathways can lead to improved patient satisfaction, less variation in the patient care, shorter LoS, and a reduction in complications and re-admissions. The ER model is not restricted to elective surgery; it offers the opportunity to improve the care of emergency admissions also.

Transfer of ER packages to obstetrics are feasible but will present some challenges. Enhanced recovery would fit well in the pathway for the elective caesarean section, but there is little experience incorporating support of the newborn and the establishment of breastfeeding into ER pathways.

CONCLUSION

The main elements of enhanced recovery pathways can lead to safe, high-quality surgical care of patients. More evidence of benefit is needed to support ER such that it should become standard practice for all women undergoing elective gynaecological surgery.

However, current data appears to show that ER provides opportunities to benefit both patients and the NHS through savings from decreased LoS and more rapid recovery. The key components of ER programmes within gynaecology appear to be:

- Optimising the patient physically and psychologically through preoperative assessment, planning and preparation before admission
- Reducing the physiological stress of the operation. Changing from an abdominal approach to a laparoscopic approach for hysterectomy where possible should be considered a priority for departments, reducing length of stay and short-term postoperative morbidity. Delivery of these techniques need not be expensive or require the use of robotic surgery but may require further training in laparoscopic surgical techniques
- A structured approach to peri- and postoperative management. Reducing the variation in care using ER pathways within a department leads to better patient care, less use of high dependency beds, fewer complications and reduced LoS. Staff satisfaction is also improved
- Patient involvement at every step of the process from decision to discharge makes them partners in their care. They are more informed, involved, motivated and overall have an improved experience

Key points for clinical practice

- Enhanced recovery provides safe high-quality perioperative care.
- Informed decision making about the options for treatment leads to greater patient satisfaction and reduces unnecessary surgery.
- Preoperative optimisation and day of surgery admission are key elements of enhanced recovery.
- Avoiding dehydration using free clear fluids up to 2 hours prior to surgery and the use of complex carbohydrate drinks improves the patient care and reduces postoperative nausea and length of stay.
- A minimally invasive laparoscopic or vaginal approach to hysterectomy should be used if feasible and safe, reducing the use of the abdominal approach.
- Intraoperatively hypothermia should be avoided. Goal directed fluid therapy may be beneficial for more major procedures such a major oncology debulking surgery.
- Avoid the use of packs and drains and remove catheters as early as possible.
- Postoperatively, early feeding and mobilisation leads to a quicker recovery.
- Discharge is appropriate when the following criteria are met: Control of pain with oral analgesia; passing of urine with minimal residual (or when patient can self-manage the catheter if left in situ, with a planned ward attendance for removal at a later date); passage of flatus and mobilisation. Discharge planning starts in the outpatients at the initial visit when the patient and her carers are informed of the expected length of stay.
- Enhanced recovery for the obstetric patient poses a challenge as we deal with two patients and four specialties as well as the physiology of establishing breastfeeding.

REFERENCES

1. Kehlet H. Fast-track colorectal surgery. Lancet 2008; 371:791–793.
2. Knott A, Pathak S, McGrath JS, et al. Consensus views on implementation and measurement of enhanced recovery after surgery in England: Delphi study. BMJ Open 2012; 2:e001878.
3. Kennedy AD, Sculpher MJ, Coulter A, et al. Effects of decision aids for menorrhagia on treatment choices, health outcomes and costs: a randomized controlled trial. JAMA 2002; 288:2701–2708.
4. Bottle, A, P. Aylin. Variations in vaginal and abdominal hysterectomy by region and trust in England. BJOG 2005; 112:326–328.
5. Brummer TH, Jalkanen J, Fraser J, et al. FINHYST 2006 – national prospective 1-year survey of 5,279 hysterectomies. Hum Reprod 2009; 24:2515–2522.
6. Borendal-Wodlin N, Nilsson L, Kjolhede P. Health related quality of life and post operative recovery in fast track hysterectomy. Acta Obstet Gynecol Scan 2011; 90:362–368.
7. Noblett SE, Watson DS, Huong H, et al. Pre-operative oral carbohydrate loading in colorectal surgery: a randomized controlled trial. Colorectal Dis 2006; 8:563–569.
8. Gustafsson UO, Scott MJ, Schwenk W, et al. Guidelines for perioperative care in elective colonic surgery: Enhanced Recovery After Surgery (ERAS®) Society recommendations. Clin Nutr 2012; 31:783–800.
9A. Güenaga KF, Matos D, Wille-Jørgensen P. Mechanical bowel preparation for elective colorectal surgery. Cochrane Database Syst Rev 2011; 7; :CD001544.
9B. Nieboer T, Johnson N, Lethaby A, et al. Surgical approach to hysterectomy for benign gynaecological disease. Cochrane Database Syst Rev 2010; (3):CD003677.
9C. Mäkinen J, Brummer T, Jalkanen J, et al. Ten years of progress—improved hysterectomy outcomes in Finland 1996–2006: a longitudinal observation study. BMJ Open 2013; 3:e003169.
10A. Franchi M, Trimbos J, Zanaboni F, et al. Randomised trial of drains versus no drains following radical hysterectomy and pelvic lymph node dissection: a European Organisation for Research and Treatment of Cancer-Gynaecological Cancer Group (EORTC-GCG) study in 234 patients. Eur J Cancer 2007; 43:1265–1268.
10B. Liu H, Zhang Y, Zhang Y, et al. Drain versus no-drain after gastrectomy for patients with advanced gastric cancer: systematic review and meta-analysis. Dig Surg 2011; 28:178–189.
10C. Putzu M, Casati A, Berti M, et al. Clinical complications, monitoring and management of perioperative mild hypothermia: anesthesiological features. Acta Biomed 2007; 78:163–169.
11. Chattopadhyay S, Mittal S, Christian S, et al. The role of intraoperative fluid optimization using the esophageal doppler in advanced gynecological cancer: early postoperative recovery and fitness for discharge. Int J Gynecol Cancer 2013; 23:199–207.
12. Borendal-Wodlin N, Nilsson L, Kjølhede P. The impact of mode of anaesthesia on postoperative recovery from fast-track abdominal hysterectomy: a randomised clinical trial. BJOG 2011; 118:299–308.
13. Albrecht E, Kirkham KR, Liu SS, et al. Perioperative intravenous administration of magnesium sulphate and postoperative pain: a meta-analysis. Anaesthesia 2013; 68:79–90.
14. De Oliveira GS Jr, Castro-Alves LJ, Khan JH, et al. Perioperative systemic magnesium to minimize postoperative pain: a meta-analysis of randomized controlled trials. Anesthesiology 2013; 119:178–190.
15. De Oliveira GS Jr, Agarwal D, Benzon HT. Perioperative single dose ketorolac to prevent postoperative pain: a meta-analysis of randomized trials. Anesth Analg 2012; 114:424–433.
16. Sun Y, Li T, Wang N, et al. Perioperative systemic lidocaine for postoperative analgesia and recovery after abdominal surgery: a meta-analysis of randomized controlled trials. Dis Colon Rectum 2012; 55:1183–1194.
17. Laskowski K, Stirling A, McKay WP, et al. A systematic review of intravenous ketamine for postoperative analgesia. Can J Anaesth. 2011; 58:911–923.
18. Ho KY, Gan TJ, Habib AS. Gabapentin and postoperative pain – a systematic review of randomized controlled trials. Pain 2006; ; 126:91–101.
19. Finch L, Phillips A, Acheson N, et al. An evaluation of the effects of a service change from epidurals to rectus sheath catheters on postoperative pain. J Obstet Gynaecol. 2013; 33:502–504.
20. Charoenkwan K, Phillipson G, Vutyavanich T. Early versus delayed oral fluids and food for reducing complications after major abdominal gynecologic surgery. Cochrane Database of Syst Rev 2007:CD004508.
21. Kroon UB, Radstrom M, Hjelthe C, et al. Fast track hysterectomy: a randomised controlled study. Eur J Obstet Gynecol Reprod Biol 2010; 151:203–207.
22. Acheson N, Crawford R. Commentary. The impact of mode of anaesthesia on post-operative recovery from fast track abdominal hysterectomy: a randomised clinical trial. BJOG 2011; 118:271–273.

23. Carter J. Szabo R. Sim WW, et al. Fast track surgery: a clinical audit. Aust N Z J Obstet Gynaecol 2010; 50:159–163.
24. Chase DM, Lopez S, Nguyen CN, et al. A clinical pathway for postoperative management and early patient discharge, does it work in gynecologic oncology? Am J Obstet Gynecol 2008; 199:541.e1–7.
25. Kalogera E, Bakkum-Gamez JN, Jankowski CJ, et al. Enhanced recovery in gynecologic surgery. Obstet Gynecol 2013; 122:319–328.
26. Lv D, Wang X, Shi G. Perioperative enhanced recovery programmes for gynaecological cancer patients. Cochrane Database of Syst Rev 2010; 16:CD008239.
27. Esnaola NF, Cole DJ. Perioperative normothermia during major surgery: is it important? Adv Surg 2011; 45:249–263.
28. Sjetne IS, Krogstad U, Ødegård S, et al. Improving quality by introducing enhanced recovery after surgery in a gynaecological department: consequences for ward nursing practice. Qual Saf Health Care 2009; 18:236–240.

Chapter 3

Contemporary diagnosis and treatment of heavy menstrual bleeding

Natalie AM Cooper, T Justin Clark

INTRODUCTION

When considering 'contemporary' practice we think of up-to-date, current and even novel practice. Current management of heavy menstrual bleeding (HMB) is eclectic. There is guidance regarding the management of HMB [1], but it mainly focuses on treatment, without giving clear advice on how best to investigate women with HMB. Clinicians are left to decide what investigative tests they will perform and in what setting, dependent upon the resources available to them and their own skills and preferences. It is only when a correct diagnosis has been made that clinicians can instigate appropriate treatment with the best chance of optimising clinical outcome. Thus, accurate diagnosis is of key importance for the successful management of HMB. In addition to diagnosis there have been developments in the treatment of HMB. Advances in therapeutic health technologies have impacted upon the type and setting of treatment. Furthermore, recent evidence from primary and secondary research has provided valuable effectiveness data on which to guide and increasingly standardise practice for the management of HMB. This chapter will examine how clinical diagnosis and treatment of heavy menstrual bleeding has evolved over recent years.

What is heavy menstrual bleeding?

Heavy menstrual bleeding is menstruation at regular intervals but with excessive flow and duration. Quantitatively, menstruation is considered heavy when menstrual loss is in excess of 80 mL [2]. It is thought to affect 1 in 5 women and leads to a third of gynaecological referrals from general practitioners [3]. However, quantifying menstrual blood loss is of limited value in the clinical setting as it is does not represent the adverse effect on health related quality of life. In addition, measuring menstrual blood loss is impractical in a clinical setting and so tends to be restricted to research settings. A more valuable definition of HMB, used by the National Institute for Clinical Excellence (NICE)

Natalie AM Cooper MBChB, PhD Women's Health Research Unit, The Blizard Institute, Barts and The London School of Medicine and Dentistry, London, UK. Email: natalie.cooper@qmul.ac.uk (for correspondence)

T Justin Clark MBChB MRCOG MD, University of Birmingham, Birmingham Women's Hospital, Birmingham, UK.

is 'excessive menstrual blood loss which interferes with the woman's physical, emotional, social and material quality of life, and which can occur alone or in combination with other symptoms [1]'. This definition considers how all aspects of a woman's wellbeing can be adversely affected by HMB and it reflects the symptoms that patients complain of.

Causes of heavy menstrual bleeding

There are a variety of causes of HMB which are detailed in **Table 3.1**. In the majority of patients the pathology associated with HMB is benign but a small number of patients (<5%) will have premalignant or malignant [6] disease, although these diagnoses are more common in women over the age of 45 years. Therefore, NICE recommend that an endometrial biopsy (EB) should be taken in women over the age of 45 years or where there is clinical suspicion of malignant or premalignant condition [1].

A classification system has also been recently accepted by the International Federation of Gynaecology and Obstetrics (FIGO) for causes of abnormal uterine bleeding in the reproductive years. This system, based on the acronym PALM-COEIN (polyps, adenomyosis, leiomyoma, malignancy and hyperplasia-coagulopathy, ovulatory disorders, endometrial causes, iatrogenic, not classified) was developed to aid the conduct and interpretation of research into abnormal uterine bleeding (AUB) [7].

INVESTIGATION OF HEAVY MENSTRUAL BLEEDING

Contemporary tests for evaluating the uterus include transvaginal scan (TVS), saline infusion sonography (SIS), outpatient hysteroscopy (OPH) and global endometrial biopsy (**Table 3.2**). Recent changes in the diagnostic work up of HMB have focused on its delivery and clinical setting. Traditional consultations take place in outpatient clinics where clinicians have limited access to real time outpatient testing. Consequently, the

Table 3.1 Causes of heavy menstrual bleeding	
Cause	Definition
Dysfunctional uterine bleeding	Irregular or excessive uterine bleeding in the absence of pregnancy, infection, trauma, new growth or hormone treatment (i.e. absence of identifiable organic pathology) [1]
Uterine fibroids	Smooth-muscle tumours of the uterus, generally benign although occasionally (<1%) malignant. Vary greatly in size from millimetres to tens of centimetres. Associated with heavy periods, pressure symptoms and occasionally pain. Fibroids respond to oestrogen and progesterone and thus tend to shrink after the menopause [1]
Endometrial pathology: Polyps	Focal outgrowths occuring anywhere within the uterine cavity. Contain variable amount of glandular tissue, stroma and blood vessels. The relative amounts of these tissue components influence their macroscopic appearance. Most polyps are benign (>99%) [4]
Hyperplasia	Proliferation of endometrial glands with structural abnormalities and crowding. Atypical hyperplasia is a proliferation of glands exhibiting cytological atypia in the nuclei and is considered pre-malignant [5]
Cancer	Well-differentiated carcinoma distinguished from atypical hyperplasia by presence of endometrial stromal invasion. Cancer is rare in premenopausal women [5]

Table 3.2 Description of currently used tests for the diagnosis of uterine pathology		
Test	Description	Diagnostic capability
Detecting structural abnormalities		
Transvaginal ultrasound (TVS)	The ultrasound transducer (probe) is inserted into the vagina and is closer to pelvic structures than in conventional transabdominal ultrasound	Endometrial, focal (polyps, submucous fibroids, other intracavity), myometrial (adenomyosis, fibroids) and adnexal pathology
Saline infusion ultrasound	Sterile saline is injected via a small cervical catheter during transvaginal ultrasonography, allowing real-time imaging of the uterus as saline fills and distends the endometrial cavity, visualising anatomical structures	As for TVS but with enhanced diagnosis of intrauterine pathology
Outpatient hysteroscopy	Direct visualisation of the inside of the uterus by passing a hysteroscope into the uterus via the vagina and cervix. During the procedure a biopsy may be taken	Endometrial and focal pathology (polyps, submucous fibroids, other intracavity) pathology
Detecting histological abnormalities		
Endometrial biopsy	The endometrium is sampled 'blindly', passing a sampler through the cervix and employing suction to obtain endometrial tissue for histological analysis	Endometrial diseases (endometrial hyperplasia with or without cytological atypia and endometrial carcinoma)

doctor and patient interaction is restricted to history taking and clinical examination with no possibility of conducting investigative tests to help confirm the diagnosis during that appointment. Global endometrial biopsy can be undertaken when clinically indicated, but patients would still need to return for the results once the sample had been processed and examined by a pathologist. It is common for patients to be sent home to await an appointment for an ultrasound scan and then be reviewed back in clinic with the results. This conventional 'multi-stop' approach ultimately results in a delay in initiating treatment of HMB. An alternative, contemporary model of care is the 'one-stop' ambulatory clinic, where the clinician sees the patient in a setting where investigations can be performed and treatments started at that appointment, if appropriate. This approach has potential benefits to patients, doctors and the wider health service.

Patients value the immediacy of care; the convenience of real time diagnosis avoids unnecessary delay minimising anxiety and the inconvenience and costs associated with scheduled follow up appointments [8]. Treatment options can be discussed and in some circumstances treatment can be initiated at first contact reducing morbidity from on-going untreated HMB. Examples of such therapeutic interventions include fitting of the levonorgesterol-releasing intrauterine system (LNG-IUS – Mirena) or undertaking minor hysteroscopic surgery to remove polyps and small fibroids [9–11]. Where simultaneous diagnosis and treatment is not possible or desired, management plans can be formulated based upon the diagnostic assessment, e.g. grading of submucous fibroids and planning the best technique, setting and preparation for hysteroscopic myomectomy or determining the suitability and likely outcomes of endometrial ablation based upon the cavity shape and dimensions. Whilst there may be psychological and clinical benefits from minimising delay in diagnosis and treatment, it is possible that patients may experience increased levels of anxiety when attending more interventional 'see and treat' clinics compared with conventional general outpatient departments. One study evaluating an ambulatory one stop hysteroscopy clinic supports this contention but it found that the levels of anxiety were comparable to women attending pelvic pain clinics and lower than those for women attending for colposcopy [12]. The same study also found that women were satisfied with the outpatient procedure and that the outpatient setting was not associated with dissatisfaction [12].

A seamless approach to managing HMB is potentially advantageous to health care professionals and health services. This is because the efficiency of diagnosis and treatment is enhanced and resource use associated with the need for repeated outpatient follow up is avoided. Service capacity, especially that relating to expensive operating theatre resource and scarce inpatient hospital beds, is also substantially increased. However, these significant, prospective economic benefits of integrated outpatient diagnostic and treatment services in HMB may be offset by other inherent service requirements. These include prolongation of the appointment times required to allow one or a combination of TVS, SIS or OPH to be performed during the consultation, such that fewer patients can be seen during a clinical session. Additional economic considerations include the capital outlay needed to support the development and maintenance of necessary infrastructure, equipment and competency.

Cost-effectiveness of diagnosis in heavy menstrual bleeding

A recent cost-effectiveness study has examined the use of the four main diagnostic tests (TVS, EB, OPH and SIS) used for investigation of HMB [13]. The four testing modalities were looked at to determine which was the most cost-effective test or combination of tests for investigating women with HMB in a contemporary 'one-stop' setting. These strategies were compared to a strategy of 'no investigation' where women were not investigated but instead were immediately treated with a LNG-IUS. Five possible causes of HMB were considered (i) intracavity lesions (polyps and submucous fibroids), (ii) small intramural fibroids (uterus <12 weeks size), (iii) large intramural fibroids (uterus >12 weeks size), (iv) endometrial disease (subdivided into complex hyperplasia and complex hyperplasia with atypia or endometrial cancer) and (v) dysfunctional uterine bleeding (DUB). These underlying pathologies were allocated a specific treatment, predefined by an expert clinical panel, to ensure that decision making was consistent. Small intramural fibroids, complex hyperplasia and DUB were all treated with the LNG-IUS; large intramural fibroids and complex hyperplasia with atypia or endometrial cancer were treated with hysterectomy and intracavity lesions were treated by hysteroscopic removal. The model assumed that where a diagnosis could be made at the initial appointment, treatments such as the LNG-IUS and hysteroscopic removal of polyps would be undertaken concurrently. The only exception to this 'see and treat' approach was for the model based upon initial testing with EB alone, because treatment could not be initiated until the histology results became available.

The base case cost-effectiveness model was founded upon a population of women aged 45 years and without future fertility desires in keeping with the more prevalent demographic of women presenting to secondary care with HMB [14]. The clinical outcome measure used in the model was cost per patient satisfied. This measure was chosen because it is the most widely used outcome reported in the published literature and the perception of HMB is based on patients' subjective assessment of their bleeding symptoms. The presumption was that if a test or testing strategy was accurate for diagnosing a particular pathology associated with HMB, appropriate treatment could be instigated, optimising clinical outcome, i.e. level of satisfaction. Patients who were dissatisfied after their first treatment, either because of the intrinsic limitations of available treatments or an incorrect initial diagnosis, were given a second line treatment.

Data regarding disease prevalence, test success and accuracy and patient satisfaction with treatment were taken from the published literature when possible. Systematic reviews with meta-analysis were considered the highest quality and data from this type of study were used when possible. When data could not be identified from the literature an expert panel were surveyed for their opinions regarding the clinical scenario. Costs were taken from department of health, healthcare resource group (HRG) codes.

The results of the cost-effectiveness study were that outpatient hysteroscopy or outpatient hysteroscopy combined with endometrial biopsy were the most cost-effective options when compared to immediate treatment with the LNG-IUS. The decision between the two diagnostic options depends upon how much the health care provider, in this case the NHS, are willing to pay to gain an additional patient who is satisfied after treatment. Diagnostic work up based upon OPH alone was estimated from the analytical modelling to cost an additional £359 to gain one extra woman satisfied over treatment alone with LNG-IUS. A combination of outpatient hysteroscopy and endometrial biopsy cost an additional £21,500 to gain an extra woman satisfied. Although patient reported outcomes such as cost per satisfied patient, are not directly equitable to cost utility outcomes, i.e. additional cost per quality adjusted life year (QALY) gained, the additional costs fall within the level used for cost per QALY, where NICE would consider it affordable to the NHS (£20,000 –£30,000 threshold) [15].

The cost-effectiveness model was also adapted to reflect a population who wanted to retain fertility and also to reflect the scenario recommended by NICE, in which women with HMB should have had initial treatment with a LNG-IUS fitted in primary care and are only referred to a gynaecologist if they do not respond to treatment [1]. In both of these adapted strategies, an initial testing strategy of OPH alone was found to be the most cost-effective option. To allow for comparison with the traditional delivery of HMB services, the economic model was adapted a third time to reflect conventional patient care encompassing multiple visits. All of the treatments strategies in this model were more expensive than in the 'one-stop' models. This analysis found that initial testing with SIS alone or a combination of OPH and EB were the cost-effective options.

Thus, OPH with or without EB appears to be the preferred option for investigating women, no matter what their presentation to secondary care is, nor which model of clinical care is followed. Inevitably with any economic modelling exercise simplifications and assumptions have to be made such that not all aspects of testing can be captured. For example, a disadvantage of OPH compared with pelvic ultrasound is that it does not image the myometrium, adnexae or pelvis. Although asymptomatic ovarian or adnexal pathology requiring treatment is rarely found during investigations for HMB [16], women may feel reassured when they know that these structures have been examined and are normal. Furthermore, this economic model used the tariffs allocated to treatment by HRGs rather than bottom-up costing, and so may not be an accurate reflection of the true costs to the health service. Moreover, the NHS perspective of the economic analysis may have underestimated the total cost savings of one-stop service delivery had a wider social perspective been considered. Minimising interference to women's home and working lives by avoiding unnecessary follow-up appointments, with consequent travel and waiting times is likely to be associated with substantial economic benefits. If the absence from paid work and household activities had been quantified in monetary units, these costs may have also been significant. Thus, it is probable that a one-stop setting for investigation of

HMB from a societal view point would have been even more cost-effective compared with traditional multi-stop models of service delivery.

Training and setting

Expanding provision of contemporary ambulatory diagnostic and treatment services for common gynaecological conditions such as HMB will require training of health care professionals both conducting and supporting procedures. Gynaecologists and nurse specialists [17] will need to gain competency in core craft skills such as gynaecological scanning, outpatient hysteroscopy and minor outpatient surgery. Training programmes will need to adapt to ensure relevant proficiencies. The minimally invasive nature of current outpatient testing for uterine and pelvic evaluation combined with the miniaturisation and increasing portability of diagnostic technologies means that such interventions need be restricted to the hospital environment. Delivery of diagnostic and therapeutic services in HMB can be delivered in the community by gynaecologists and specialist general practitioners or nurses.

TREATMENT OF HEAVY MENSTRUAL BLEEDING

Medical treatment

For DUB, the LNG-IUS is recommended by NICE as the first-line medical treatment [1]. The ECLIPSE study is a recently published multicentre randomised controlled trial (RCT) which compared the LNG-IUS to usual medical therapy for treatment of HMB in primary care [20]. Women who were randomised to LNG-IUS were twice as likely to have continued with the treatments as those women who were randomised to usual medical therapy after 2 years. Women in the both groups reported that their bleeding was improved, however the improvement observed in the LNG-IUS group was significantly greater at 6, 12 and 24 months. This study also showed that women with a BMI >25 were more likely to have improved bleeding with the LNG-IUS than with usual medical therapy, presumably because absorption is better. Quality of life was improved in both groups, without any significant difference between the groups.

Another recent area of development in the medical treatment of HMB has been the development of the selective progesterone receptor modulator, ulipristal acetate. Two RCTs have been published showing its short-term safety and effectiveness for the pretreatment of fibroids associated with HMB prior to surgery. The drug is licensed for up to two intermittent courses of 3-month treatment and there remain concerns over its long-term safety especially as regards its effect on the endometrium where non-physiological changes have been observed although these appear to be reversible following cessation of use [21–22]. The high rates of amenorrhoea and resolution of HMB observed suggest that this group of drugs have the potential to provide future, effective medical treatments for HMB and fibroids.

Hysteroscopic surgery

Endoscopic instrumentation and associated technologies have developed over recent years increasing the feasibility and widening the repertoire of hysteroscopic and other intrauterine surgery in women with HMB. Miniaturisation of hysteroscopic systems has established hysteroscopy as an outpatient diagnostic tool. Moreover, developments in mechanical and electrosurgical ancillary instruments have facilitated the removal of acquired intrauterine pathologies such as polyps and small fibroids in an outpatient setting at the time of diagnosis. Fragile mechanical hysteroscopic instruments have been superseded by bipolar electrodes (Versapoint) to resect these focal lesions [9–11]. Newly developed morcellators and bipolar resectoscopes offer alternative methods for removing polyps and fibroids, allowing large and multiple intrauterine pathologies to be removed [11]. These technologies are suitable for use in physiological saline. Thus, there is the potential to improve the feasibility and safety of advanced hysteroscopic surgery such as hysteroscopic myomectomy.

Endometrial ablation

Rapid, semi-automated ablative devices to treat HMB are well-established. The effectiveness of these so-called 'second generation' ablative technologies is comparable to first generation hysteroscopic techniques. A recent meta-analysis of individual patient data (IPD) showed no significant difference between rates of dissatisfaction associated with first and second generation approaches respectively (12% and 11%). Factors were identified that were associated with reduced dissatisfaction when undertaking second generation endometrial ablation and these included uterine sound lengths ≤8 cm and absence of fibroids or polyps [23]. Older age (over 45 years) also appears to be associated with better clinical outcomes from a recent interrogation of hospital episode statistics (HES) database [24]. These findings should be considered when counselling patients and formulating management plans. When the LNG-IUS was compared with endometrial destruction techniques no significant difference in dissatisfaction rates was identified [23]. These findings support NICEs recommendation that endometrial ablation can be offered in place of LNG-IUS when patients have contraindications, or do not want hormonal treatment [1], given that the two treatments have comparable outcomes. A head-to-head RCT comparing the LNG-IUS with endometrial ablation (the MIRA trial) is underway in the Netherlands and may inform practice further in due course.

Over recent years these endometrial ablative technologies have been demonstrated to be feasible, acceptable and effective when used in an ambulatory setting with suitable local anaesthesia [25–26].

Hysterectomy

A recently published IPD meta-analysis has suggested that treatment of HMB with hysterectomy results in the lowest levels of dissatisfaction when compared to endometrial destruction techniques and LNG-IUS [23]. However, dissatisfaction was low for all of the treatments at 12 months follow-up. When hysterectomy was compared to first generation endometrial destruction, the dissatisfaction rates were 5% and 13% respectively and this difference was statistically significant ($P<0.001$). When hysterectomy was indirectly compared to the LNG-IUS (direct comparisons were not possible with the retrieved data) the rates were 5% and 17%, although this was not statistically significant ($P = 0.07$). Hysterectomy was considered the most cost-effective treatment for HMB; however, the cost-effectiveness analysis used a long-term end-point of 10 years [27].

Despite the apparent longer term economic benefits of hysterectomy, the procedure removes future fertility and is invasive being associated with significant morbidity and prolonged recovery. These considerations preclude its use as a first-line treatment for HMB, unless premalignant atypical hyperplasia or cancer has been diagnosed or large fibroids are detected, contraindicating the LNG-IUS or endoscopic interventions, in women not requiring their fertility. However, advances in laparoscopic surgical techniques and technologies, especially advanced bipolar electrosurgical instruments and ultrasonic energy modalities, have facilitated minimally invasive hysterectomy. Day case hysterectomy (patients discharged <24 hours after surgery) is being performed in some centres [28] and a RCT (HEALTH trial) is due to start shortly comparing laparoscopic subtotal hysterectomy with endometrial ablation. Thus, in time the place of hysterectomy in the treatment of HMB will need to be reassessed. This evolution in care has in part been driven by enhanced recovery programmes which are associated with reduced costs due to shorter hospital stay and benefits to the patient such as reduced risk of venous thromboembolic events and hospital acquired infections [29].

CONCLUSION

Heavy menstrual bleeding remains one of the commonest presenting complaints in gynaecology. Diagnosis of the potential causes of HMB is of prime importance in order to provide optimal treatment. Technological advances, especially in imaging and endoscopic instrumentation have facilitated outpatient diagnosis and treatment. The outpatient or 'ambulatory' one-stop model of care appears to confer advantages over traditional models in terms of cost and patient satisfaction. Evidence supports the use of the LNG-IUS as the first line medical treatment for HMB, particularly as it can be fitted conveniently in primary care. Hysterectomy remains an effective treatment option for HMB refractory to medical or less invasive surgical interventions such as endometrial ablation. Indeed, the long-term clinical and economic benefits of hysterectomy over the LNG-IUS and endometrial ablation may support its first line use in some circumstances. In time, the place of hysterectomy for the treatment of HMB may need to be reassessed with the increasing use of less invasive methods for conducting hysterectomy and quicker return to normal functioning with the adoption of enhanced recovery programmes.

Key points for clinical practice

- Traditional models of care which involve patients attending multiple clinic appointments cause delays in patient care as well as increased levels of anxiety.
- One-stop investigation and management of heavy menstrual bleeding is acceptable to patients and is likely to be more cost-effective.
- Training will need to adapt to accommodate the shift towards clinicians performing their own investigations in a one-stop setting.
- The majority of women who present with heavy menstrual bleeding can be treated in the outpatient setting either with a levonorgestrel intrauterine system, endometrial ablation or removal of intracavity lesions.
- The levonorgestrel intrauterine system is the most effective medical therapy for the treatment of heavy menstrual bleeding, particularly in women with a raised body mass index.
- When assessing long-term benefit, hysterectomy is associated with lower dissatisfaction levels than the levonorgestrel intrauterine system. Day case hysterectomy is becoming a reality and may further support hysterectomy being considered as a possible first-line option for heavy menstrual bleeding.

REFERENCES

1. National Institute for Clinical Excellence (NICE). CG44 Heavy menstrual bleeding. London: NICE, 2007.
2. Hallberg L. Nilsson L. Determination of menstrual blood loss. Sca J Clin Lab Invest 1964; 16:244–228.
3. Coulter A, Noone A, Goldacre M. General practitioners' referrals to specialist outpatient clinics. I. Why general practitioners refer patients to specialist outpatient clinics. Br Med J 1989 ; 299:304.
4. Clark TJ, Gupta JK. Handbook of Outpatient Hysteroscopy. A complete guide to diagnosis and therapy. London: Hodder Education; 2005.
5. Kurman RJ, Kaminski PF, Norris HJ. The behavior of endometrial hyperplasia. A long-term study of 'untreated' hyperplasia In 170 patients. Cancer 1985; 56:403–412.
6. Iram S, Musonda P, Ewies AA. Premenopausal bleeding: when should the endometrium be investigated? A retrospective non-comparative study of 3006 women. Eur J Obstet Gynecol Reprod Biol 2010; 148:86–89.
7. Munro MG, Critchley HO, Fraser IS. The FIGO systems for nomenclature and classification of causes of abnormal uterine bleeding in the reproductive years: who needs them? Am J Obstet Gynecol 2012; 207:259–265.
8. Maiti S, Naidoo K. Patients' satisfaction survey at the outpatient hysteroscopy service at St. Mary's hospital, Manchester, UK. Menopause Int 2008; 14:4 188-192.
9. Capobianco G, Vargiu N, Dessole F, et al. Office hysteroscopy for uterine intracavitary pathologies: see and treat approach. Gynecological Surg 2009; 6:1 supplement, 72.
10. Farrugia M, McMillan L. Versapoint (TM) in the treatment of focal intra-uterine pathology in an outpatient clinic setting. Ref Gynecol Obstet 2000; 7:169–173.
11. Emanuel MH, Wamsteker K. The Intra Uterine Morcellator: a new hysteroscopic operating technique to remove intrauterine polyps and myomas. J Minim Invasive Gynecol. 2005; 12:62–66.
12. Gupta JK, Clark TJ, More S, et al. Patient anxiety and experiences associated with an outpatient 'one-stop' 'see and treat' hysteroscopy clinic. Surg Endosc. 2004; 18:1099–1104.
13. Cooper NA, Barton PM, Breijer M, et al. Cost-effectiveness of diagnostic strategies for the management of abnormal uterine bleeding (heavy menstrual bleeding and post-menopausal bleeding): a decision analysis. Health Technol Assess 2014; 18:1-202.
14. Higham JM, Shaw RW. Clinical associations with objective menstrual blood volume. Eur J Obstet Gynecol Reprod Biol 1999; 82:73–76.
15. National Institute for Clinical Excellence (NICE). Guide to the methods of technology appraisal 2013. London: NICE, 2013.
16. Jones K, Bourne T. The feasibility of a 'one stop' ultrasound-based clinic for the diagnosis and management of abnormal uterine bleeding. Ultrasound ObstetGynecol 2001; 17:517–521.
17. Ludkin H, Quinn P, Jones SE, et al. The benefits of setting up a nurse hysteroscopy service. Prof Nurse 2003; 19:220–222.
20. Gupta J, Kai J, Middleton L, et al. Levonorgestrel intrauterine system versus medical therapy for menorrhagia. N Eng J Med 2013; 368:128–137.
21. Donnez J, Tomaszewski J, Vázquez F, et al. Ulipristal acetate versus leuprolide acetate for uterine fibroids. N Engl J Med. 2012; 366:421–432.
22. Donnez J, Tatarchuk TF, Bouchard P, et al. Ulipristal acetate versus placebo for fibroid treatment before surgery. N Engl J Med 2012; 366:409–420.
23. Middleton LJ, Champaneria R, Daniels JP, et al. Hysterectomy, endometrial destruction, and levonorgestrel releasing intrauterine system (Mirena) for heavy menstrual bleeding: Systematic review and meta-analysis of data from individual patients. Br Med J 2010; 341 c3929.
24. Bansi-Matharu L, Gurol-Urganci I, Mahmood T, et al. Rates of subsequent surgery following endometrial ablation among English women with menorrhagia: population-based cohort study. Br J Obs Gynaecol 2013; 120:1500–1507.
25. Daniels JP, Middleton LJ, Champaneria R, et al. Second generation endometrial ablation techniques for heavy menstrual bleeding: network meta-analysis. Br Med J (Clinical research ed) 2012; 344 e.2564.
26. Clark TJ, Samuel N, Malick S, et al. Bipolar radiofrequency compared with thermal balloon endometrial ablation in the office: a randomized controlled trial. Obstet Gynecol 2011; 117: 109-118.
27. Roberts TE, Tsourapas A, Middleton LJ, et al. Hysterectomy, endometrial ablation, and levonorgestrel releasing intrauterine system (Mirena) for treatment of heavy menstrual bleeding: cost effectiveness analysis. Br Med J (Clinical research ed) 2011; 34 d2201.
28. Torbe E, Louden K. An enhanced recovery programme for women undergoing hysterectomy. Int J Gynecol Obstet 2012; 119 s690.
29. Bell A, Relph S, Sivashanmugarajan V, et al. Enhanced recovery programmes: do these have a role in gynaecology? J Obstet Gynaecol 2013; 33:539–541.

Chapter 4

Management of tubal ectopic pregnancy

Amelia Davison, Jackie A Ross

INTRODUCTION

Ectopic pregnancy is defined as the implantation of a fertilised ovum outside of the endometrial cavity, most commonly in the fallopian tube. Ectopic pregnancy is a common problem with a reported incidence of 1–2% and a UK prevalence of nearly 12,000 diagnosed each year. The incidence of ectopic is increasing and is thought to be related to; increasing maternal age, tubal surgery, pelvic inflammatory disease and assisted reproductive techniques and perhaps most importantly, increased ascertainment [1].

Historically ectopic pregnancies were managed as life-threatening events after tubal rupture; however with modern management the majority are diagnosed early in the natural history of the condition frequently in completely asymptomatic women [2]. Ectopic pregnancy is the 5th most common cause of death according to the most recent triennial report and the most common cause of death in the first trimester [3]. Although thankfully still rare, cases of serious adverse outcomes are typically a result of delayed diagnoses or misdiagnosis. However, the mainstay of modern management of ectopic pregnancy involves early and accurate diagnosis which maximises the treatment options in clinically stable women [4].

So how were ectopics diagnosed in the past? Traditionally diagnosis was made at laparotomy with a 20% false preoperative diagnosis of a ruptured ectopic; diagnosing an unruptured ectopic was practically impossible. During the 1960s laparoscopies became popular for diagnosis, although treatment remained by means of laparotomy. In the 1980s, the first cohort study on the use of transabdominal ultrasound (TAS) to diagnose ectopic pregnancy was published. Over recent decades transvaginal ultrasound scanning (TVS) has become the imaging modality of choice for diagnosis. Transvaginal ultrasound has the advantage of an increased potential to diagnose both intrauterine pregnancies and the majority of ectopic pregnancies [2]. Historically, the combination of pelvic pain, a period of amenorrhoea and the absence of an obvious intrauterine pregnancy on TAS was accepted as an indication for diagnostic laparoscopy. In current clinical practice, how many laparoscopies are performed for the sole purpose of obtaining a diagnosis, and

Amelia Davison MRCOG, Early Pregnancy and Gynaecology Assessment Unit, King's College Hospital, London UK.

Jackie A Ross FRCOG, Early Pregnancy and Gynaecology Assessment Unit, King's College Hospital, London, UK.
Email: jackie.ross1@nhs.net (for correspondence)

how many laparotomies do we now undertake to treat an ectopic pregnancy? The answer is hopefully very few. This is due to a number of key developments in early pregnancy care. Firstly, the use of highly sensitive urinary pregnancy tests, detecting β-human chorionic gonadotropin (β-hCG) levels as low as 15 IU/L, enabling women to confirm their pregnancies very early, even before a menstrual period has been missed. Secondly, the setting up of early pregnancy units (EPUs) to facilitate access to dedicated ultrasound and clinical assessment.

DIAGNOSIS

The majority of ectopic pregnancies will be located in the fallopian tubes, but nontubal locations account for 5–7% of ectopic pregnancies and include interstitial, cornual, cervical, caesarean scar, ovarian and abdominal pregnancies.

Clinical

As with most medical conditions, the suspicion of an ectopic pregnancy should be raised from the clinical history. A meta-analysis has identified four strongly associated risk factors from the history including: previous ectopic pregnancy, previous tubal surgery, evidence of tubal pathology and in-utero exposure to diethylstilboestrol [5]. The clinical presentation however varies, and can be misleading with some women unsure of their last menstrual period, 10–20% presenting with no symptoms and abdominal pain often featuring as a late presentation. Clinicians should be aware of the risk of a ruptured or leaking ectopic pregnancy in any woman of reproductive age with sudden onset gastrointestinal symptoms [3].

Traditionally bimanual and speculum examinations were performed on all women attending in the acute setting but observational studies suggest that it is more important to perform an ultrasound scan. However, vaginal examination still has a role where there is no recourse to a timely ultrasound scan and a clinical decision needs to be made regarding the need for emergency surgery, or where the clinical picture and the ultrasound diagnosis do not correspond.

Ultrasound

Ultrasound diagnosis of an ectopic pregnancy was first described in 1969 when TAS was used with a false negative and false positive rate of around 50% [6]. Transvaginal ultrasound is a safe and accurate non-invasive tool that has been demonstrated to be an acceptable diagnostic procedure for women attending an EPU [7] and has a much higher diagnostic accuracy [8]. In addition, when only one scan is used to diagnose an ectopic pregnancy, ultrasound is also extremely cost effective. Recent studies have reported a 94–97% positive predictive value for TVS, with a low false positive rate, sensitivity rates of around 87–99% and specificity rates of 94–99% [9]. TVS is now an essential first line tool in diagnosing an ectopic pregnancy. So what do we expect to see at ultrasound if we are not merely reporting on the negative finding of an 'empty uterus'? Modern management involves the positive identification of an adnexal mass. Appearances have been extensively described and range from an inhomogeneous adnexal mass to an extra uterine gestational sac with a yolk sac and/or a fetal pole with or without cardiac activity (**Figure 4.1**). The location within the tube varies, but most ectopic pregnancies will be located in the ampullary region of the tube, so are seen above and medial to the ovary and two thirds are ipsilateral to the corpus luteum [10]. The whole of the adnexa should be examined to be sure not to miss the less

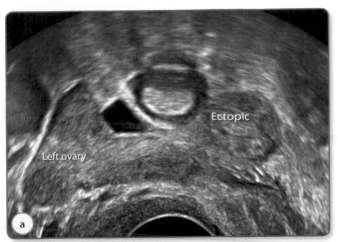

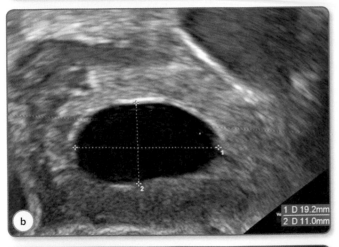

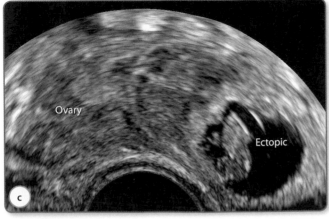

Figure 4.1 Ultrasound appearances of tubal ectopic pregnancies (a) solid ectopic (b) empty gestational sac (c) live ectopic.

common tubal locations; fimbrial ectopics are located below the ovary, and isthmic ones very high in the pelvis close to the tubal insertion [6, 11].

There are additional ultrasound findings that should point the examiner to hunt for an ectopic pregnancy. The presence of an intact endometrial echo (i.e. a tri-laminar midline echo typical of the proliferative phase of the cycle) with a history of vaginal bleeding is a highly specific indicator of ectopic pregnancy, though this finding is only seen in about two thirds of ectopic pregnancies [12]. The presence of blood in the endometrial cavity, otherwise known as a 'pseudosac' is found on TAS in up to 20% of women diagnosed with ectopic pregnancies [13]. Fluid within the pouch of Douglas is present in 10–25% of women with an ectopic pregnancy and may be either anechoic (i.e. physiological) or contain low level echoes typical of blood. Clotted blood appears solid and echogenic, similar to bowel. The presence of echogenic fluid is highly sensitive and specific for diagnosing a haemoperitoneum and so is typical of a ruptured or leaking ectopic pregnancy, but may also be due to haemorrhage from the corpus luteum or an incomplete miscarriage [14]. The amount of blood in the pelvis can be estimated on ultrasound [15]. It may be described according to how far up the posterior aspect of an anteverted uterus the fluid extends; a small amount being below the isthmus, a moderate amount up to the body of the uterus and a large amount above the fundus. If blood is visualised anterior to the uterus, an additional TAS should be done to evaluate Morison's pouch. This is the anatomical space located between the right kidney and the capsule of the liver. If blood is seen here in the supine position, then this equates to approximately 700 mL of blood in the peritoneal cavity [16]. From these additional features it is clear that ultrasound is not only used to diagnose an ectopic pregnancy but also to help determine the most appropriate management in stable patients.

A systematic approach to the examination of the pelvis during a TVS is paramount. It has been reported that the majority of women referred with suspected ectopic pregnancies to a tertiary level EPU for a second opinion, have intrauterine pregnancies that were either missed on ultrasound examination or misinterpreted as ectopic [6]. Scans should be systematically performed by skilled individuals to enable the diagnosis of the vast majority of ectopic pregnancies on the initial ultrasound scan. Recent studies have demonstrated that approximately 75% of ectopic pregnancies will be diagnosed at the initial scan and that overall the pregnancy will be located in 90% of women [9]. The uterus and cervix should be visualised in the longitudinal and transverse sections, visualising the interstitial portions of the tubes. The ovaries and adnexae need to be examined in all cases, not just those where there is the suspicion of an ectopic pregnancy. The side and number of corpora lutei should be identified and recorded. Finally, the pouch of Douglas should be examined for the type and amount of any fluid collected behind the uterus. This systematic and thorough examination will ensure that the operator becomes skilled at recognising the limits of the endometrial cavity, corpus luteum, the presence of multiple corpora lutei, fimbrial cysts, blood clots and loops of bowel, all which to the unskilled eye can be misinterpreted as an ectopic pregnancy.

Biochemistry

Considered in isolation, serum β-hCG and progesterone have no role in locating a pregnancy. Neither should the absolute β-hCG level be used to decide who to scan. This is because, the majority of women with ectopic pregnancies will have serum β-hCG levels lower than 1500 IU/L and women with ectopic pregnancies and falling or low β-hCG levels may still experience tubal rupture [17]. Biochemistry is useful in women with pregnancies of unknown location (PUL) where there is no clinical need for surgical intervention, as it can be used to triage women into different follow-up protocols according to their risk of needing treatment for an ectopic pregnancy. β-hCG is produced by proliferating trophoblast and is expected to double every 1–2 days following a linear trajectory up to a level of 1000 IU/L in a normal singleton pregnancy. Progesterone is secreted by the corpus luteum and remains relatively constant. In failing pregnancies, wherever they are located, the β-hCG will typically fail to increase normally and the progesterone levels will be low. It has been proposed that triage of women with a PUL can be based on either a combination of a single progesterone measurement in conjunction with the β-hCG at presentation or on two β hCG measurements 48 hours apart (Tables 4.1 and 4.2). The progesterone measurement predicts the pattern likely to be seen with serial β-hCG measurements, so gives the advantage of being able to discharge a significant proportion of women from routine follow up appointments and minimises the workload in chasing up women who fail to attend for their repeat β-hCG at 48 hours [18]. However, a protocol based on a single progesterone level has not yet been tested in multiple centres and this option was not considered by NICE when developing their early pregnancy guideline, so their current recommendations are based on serial β-hCGs [19].

Pregnancies where the biochemistry suggests a viable, on-going pregnancy will usually be intrauterine and TVS can be used to locate the pregnancy once the β-hCG levels are predicted to be above the local unit's discriminatory level (usually 1000–2000 IU/L). Pregnancies where the β-hCG levels are declining very quickly or the progesterone level is very low, are most likely to resolve spontaneously without intervention and without the pregnancy ever being located. Those that fall in between will need more intensive follow up to clarify the diagnosis should the β-hCG levels be increasing. NICE guidance stresses that clinicians should not be encouraged to rely on biochemistry results, but should take the clinical picture as their main priority.

Surgery

The gold standard for the diagnosis of an ectopic pregnancy will always remain histological evidence of chorionic villi in the fallopian tube, however laparoscopy is not without operative risk and neither is it 100% sensitive, though the diagnostic accuracy of laparoscopy has never been formally assessed [5]. There is a risk that early tubal and more advanced non-tubal ectopic pregnancies may be missed, and that other pathology causing tubal distension, such as a haematosalpinx, endometriosis or tubal endothelial hyperplasia may be mistaken for an ectopic pregnancy [20, 21]. The majority of women should not need

Table 4.1 Protocol for the management of patients with PUL using progesterone and initial β-hCG to triage [18]			
Progesterone (nmol/L)	β-hCG (IU/L)	Likely diagnosis	Follow-up
<10	>25	Spontaneous resolution	Discharge. To return if in pain or experiencing prolonged bleeding
>10–20	>25	Failing pregnancy	Pregnancy test in 1 week, repeat β-hCG if positive
>20–60	>25	High risk of intervention	β-hCG in 2 days
>60	<1000	Normal intrauterine pregnancy	Repeat ultrasound scan when predicted β-hCG >1000 IU/L
>60	>1000	Missed ectopic pregnancy	Repeat ultrasound scan by senior examiner as soon as possible

Table 4.2 Protocol for the management of PUL using serial β-hCG to triage [19]		
β-hCG levels 48 hours apart	likely diagnosis	Follow-up
Decrease > 50%	Spontaneous resolution	Pregnancy test in 2 weeks, return to early pregnancy units (EPU) within 24 hours if positive
Between a 50% decline and a 63% rise inclusive	Uncertain	Clinical review in the EPU within 24 hours
Increase > 63%	Developing intrauterine pregnancy	Repeat scan between 7 and 14 days
Increase > 63% and β-hCG ≥ 1500 IU/L	Missed ectopic or intrauterine pregnancy	Consider an earlier scan

to be subjected to an operative procedure to make the diagnosis of an ectopic pregnancy; laparoscopy should be reserved mainly for treatment, an accurate diagnosis having been made on ultrasound preoperatively to facilitate planning of the surgical procedure [8]. Macroscopically, the tube may appear distended by trophoblastic tissue and blood, products of conception may be seen leaking from the fimbrial end of the tube or there may be evidence of tubal rupture with bleeding from the damaged tube into the pelvis.

TREATMENT

The increased sensitivity of our diagnostic tests for ectopic pregnancies has resulted in many ectopic pregnancies being diagnosed very early in their natural course and in clinically stable patients. If the diagnosis of an ectopic pregnancy is made only at the point that a woman is in severe pain or is cardiovascularly compromised, then surgical intervention with its inherent risks and possible adverse effect on fertility, is always justified. However, before the advent of modern tests, many ectopic pregnancies would have gone undiagnosed, never becoming clinically apparent without causing any harm. The aim of modern management should be to diagnose ectopic pregnancies accurately so that women can seek prompt treatment should they become symptomatic, and to try to predict which women do require active intervention to prevent tubal rupture, whilst optimising their future fertility.

Surgical treatment

Traditionally, ectopic pregnancies were not only managed but also diagnosed by laparotomy. The first surgery performed to stop fatal bleeding from an ectopic pregnancy was reported in 1849 [2]. Following this, salpingectomy via laparotomy remained the gold standard treatment for decades. It was not until the mid-1990s that laparoscopy began to replace laparotomy. As laparoscopic skills increased, stable women with ectopic pregnancies were treated by laparoscopy but laparotomies were still first line for all ruptured ectopics. Laparoscopic surgery is now the mainstay of treatment for both ruptured and non-ruptured ectopic pregnancies regardless of the gestational age. The benefits of laparoscopic surgery are reduced patient morbidity, less intraoperative blood loss, reduced pain and decreased adhesion formation [2]. It is equally as effective as laparotomy with shorter operating time and is associated with shorter hospital stays and reduced costs. Operative laparoscopy is now the gold standard as defined by the Royal College of Obstetricians and Gynaecologists for the surgical management of haemodynamically stable patients.

There is a continuing role for laparotomy in those with a large intra-abdominal bleed where rapid haemostasis is paramount or for those with a known pelvic mass, e.g. large fibroids or severe adhesions which may make access difficult for all but the most highly skilled minimal access surgeons [1].

The first reported open salpingotomy was in 1920 however, this was not undertaken with the purpose of preserving future fertility. It was not until the 1950s that salpingotomy was considered an alternative to salpingectomy for preserving fertility. This conservative surgical approach runs the risk of persistent trophoblastic tissue, with reported failure rates of 3–29% [22A]. This can lead to recurrence of clinical symptoms and the need for further treatment In women who have undergone a salpingotomy, serum β-hCG monitoring is required to identify those with on-going trophoblastic proliferation. Clearly, this conservative surgical approach is more time consuming and requires longer follow-up. Observational studies demonstrate that salpingotomy appears to be associated with higher subsequent intrauterine pregnancy rates but also higher recurrent ectopic rates of up to 9.8%. To date there has been no clear consensus on the type of surgery that should be performed, i.e. salpingotomy or salpingectomy. However, a recent multicentre randomised trial of salpingotomy versus salpingectomy for women with a normal-looking contralateral tube, showed no difference in fertility outcomes between the two groups, but with an increased risk of persistent trophoblast in the salpingotomy group [22B]. In light of these findings, the current recommendation that salpingotomy should be reserved for those women with pathology in the contralateral tube or with only one tube remaining will need to remain in unchanged [19].

Laparoscopic salpingectomy is the mainstay of surgical treatment for tubal ectopic pregnancies. It is considered preferable to remove the affected fallopian tube as completely as possible to avoid the risk of distal recurrence, as opposed to performing a partial salpingectomy [23]. This is facilitated by using excisional techniques with electrosurgical or ultrasonic instruments, rather than using a pre-formed endo-loop suture which removes a variable portion of tube. The interstitial component of the fallopian tube cannot be excised, so women should be made aware that there remains a risk of recurrent ipsilateral ectopic pregnancy in the proximal tube.

Medical treatment

Methotrexate was first introduced as a treatment option in the mid-1980s and has been adopted as the medical treatment of choice for ectopic pregnancy. Methotrexate is a folic acid antagonist which interferes with DNA synthesis and cell proliferation. It is particularly effective on highly proliferative tissues such as trophoblast. Potential side effects include stomatitis, conjunctivitis, gastroenteritis, impaired liver function, bone marrow depression and photosensitivity. Women must refrain from further pregnancies for at least 3 months following treatment due to the risk of teratogenesis. The most common side effect is abdominal pain. Treatment is successful in a reported 65–100% of cases, but patient selection is vital. Studies from the United States of America (USA) have often included women with presumed ectopic pregnancies as defined by the absence of evidence of an intrauterine pregnancy (i.e. PULs), so caution should be used when applying these results to a population of women with positively diagnosed ectopic pregnancies. Treatment criteria to optimise success with methotrexate include; a clinically stable patient, a non-viable ectopic and relatively low β-hCG level. Patients require follow-up with β-hCG monitoring to ensure an adequately declining β-hCG. In the UK, methotrexate is most commonly given systemically as a single dose intramuscular injection without folic acid (50 mg/m^2). A second dose of methotrexate is required in 3–27% of cases if the β-hCG levels do not fall by at least 15% between 4 and 7 days. If the β-hCG falls sufficiently, the β-hCG level is monitored weekly until resolution [24]. Other regimens can include local administration or a fixed multiple dose regimen alternating with folic acid [22]. Similar success rates are reported with both single and multiple dose regimens. Contraindications to methotrexate include; pelvic pain, evidence of haemoperitoneum, liver, renal or bone marrow impairment, or a coexisting viable pregnancy (i.e. heterotopic pregnancy).

The most useful prognostic indicator of successful outcome is the initial serum β-hCG, with the likelihood of success declining as the hCG increases [25]. The β-hCG trend prior to and following methotrexate administration is also correlated with outcome. Treatment failure has been reported to be increased with serum β-hCG concentrations >5000 U/L, an ectopic pregnancy on TVS >3 cm in diameter and the presence of embryonic heart activity. The current NICE guidelines recommend that medical treatment may be suitable for women with no significant pain, an unruptured ectopic pregnancy with an adnexal mass smaller than 35 mm, no visible heartbeat and no intrauterine pregnancy (as confirmed on an ultrasound scan). The guideline states that methotrexate should be used as the first line treatment if the β-hCG is less than 1500 IU/L and that women with levels between 1500 and 5000 IU/L may be offered either surgery or methotrexate [19].

Tubal rupture can occur even with a falling serum β-hCG, so the clinical picture is vital. Any woman undergoing medical management who develops abdominal pain should be rescanned to check for evidence of tubal rupture. If a unit uses methotrexate extensively, then non-intervention in women with pain without evidence of tubal rupture, is necessary to maintain high success rates. One such unit recommends non-intervention where 'free fluid' is identified on scan as long as it does not extend into the flanks, cause a drop in haematocrit or haemodynamic instability [25A]. Tubal patency studies following methotrexate have shown patency in 77–82% of cases which is similar to those after salpingotomy. Subsequent intrauterine pregnancy rates are quoted at over 80%, with recurrent ectopic pregnancy in up to 25% [25B]. The biggest risk with the use of methotrexate is its use in women falsely diagnosed with a pregnancy of unknown location (PUL) or ectopic pregnancy. Inadvertent use in an undiagnosed intrauterine pregnancy will usually lead to miscarriage or teratogenesis [26].

Expectant management

Expectant management of ectopic pregnancy has not been routinely offered even to stable patients, with its use being limited to a small sub-group of ectopic pregnancies managed by individual clinicians with varying success rates. This has been primarily because clinicians have felt the need to offer some form of intervention for ectopic pregnancy, and also because there has been a lack of selection criteria to reliably predict the likelihood of spontaneous resolution [27]. The first reported case of expectant management was in 1955, but it was not until the 1980s that it was reported that many ectopics pregnancies are self-limiting, ending in tubal abortion or reabsorption. Initial small case series reported success rates of only 7–25%. To date, over 800 cases have been reported, and studies have found that up to 63% of women are suitable for expectant management with a spontaneous resolution rate of 57–100% [28, 29]. Some of the cases included from the USA were women with PUL and no evidence of an intrauterine pregnancy at dilatation and curettage, rather than a positive diagnosis of ectopic pregnancy, so the success rates may be overestimated in these cases.

The aim with expectant management is to select those patients where the natural history of their ectopic pregnancy results in resolution rather than rupture. The evidence suggests that the best predictor of successful resolution is the initial β-hCG result. The probability of spontaneous resolution decreases the higher the initial β-hCG level. Several studies report 88–96% resolution with β-hCG levels of <200 IU/L compared to only 21–25% resolution in women with β-hCG levels of >2000 IU/L. A decision tree has been produced to help guide clinicians and patients regarding management choice and the likelihood of successful spontaneous resolution with expectant management. All clinically stable women with a non-viable ectopic pregnancy can be considered for expectant management using these analytical approaches. The likelihood of success can easily be conveyed to the patient, enabling women to make informed decisions regarding their management [27]. We use this decision tree in our EPU and we audit our figures regularly to use when counselling women (**Figure 4.2**). Once the β-hCG is declining, levels are checked weekly until <20 IU/L or the urinary pregnancy test is negative.

Expectant management potentially reduces the risk of operative morbidity, but what are the advantages of expectant management over medical treatment? The aim of medical treatment is to induce regression of the trophoblast as reflected in a decline in β-hCG

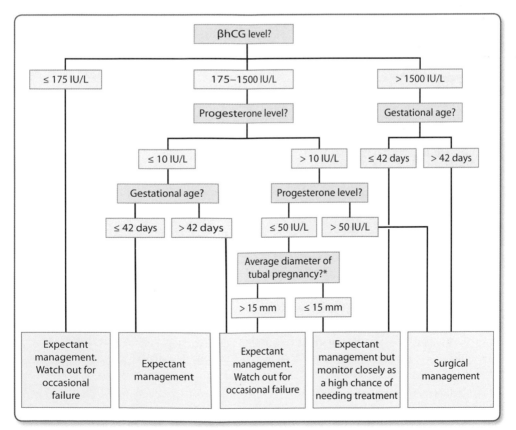

Figure 4.2 Decision tree for expectant management of tubal ectopic pregnancy. *Ectopic pregnancy diagnosed as a solid tubal mass; an extra uterine gestational sac with a yolk sac and/or a fetal pole with or without cardiac activity; an empty extra uterine gestational sac.

levels. If β-hCG is already falling, there is little to be gained by using methotrexate. If the β-hCG is relatively low (<1000 IU/L) and is plateauing or increasing very slowly, expectant management does not expose the patient to the potentially serious side effects associated with methotrexate [27]. The clinical picture can also remain clear without the 'separation pain' induced by methotrexate potentially masking the pain of leaking or impending rupture of the ectopic pregnancy. A recent randomised, unblinded study of patients with ectopic pregnancy and PUL (β-hCG <1500 and <2000 IU/L respectively), showed no difference in outcomes with expectant management versus methotrexate [30]. The results of two on-going randomised controlled trials comparing expectant management and single dose methotrexate for tubal ectopic pregnancies are awaited.

As with medical management, an expectant strategy requires a compliant, fully informed and motivated patient; one study quoted the mean time to resolution as 20 days with a range up to 67 days. Tubal rupture can occasionally occur even with low and declining β-hCG levels, so women must have means of rapid access to an emergency department and should be managed according to their clinical symptoms rather than their serum biochemistry should they become symptomatic. Long-term fertility outcomes are similar to women treated with methotrexate with several studies reporting no significant differences in fertility, intrauterine pregnancy and recurrent ectopic rates. Hysterosalpingograms in women following expectant management demonstrated tubal patency in 76% of cases and a repeat ectopic rate of 13%; comparable to the data for medical treatment [28].

CONCLUSION

The modern management of ectopic pregnancy begins with an early and accurate diagnosis achieved using sensitive β-hCG testing and skilled, high resolution TVS. The first line treatment options are now minimal access surgery, methotrexate or active monitoring. Clinicians need to balance the risk of unnecessary surgery in women with ectopic pregnancies that would have resolved without surgical intervention, against the risk of rupture with medical or expectant management. When considering the best treatment for any individual woman, this should be taken in a step-wise fashion, never forgetting that clinical symptoms and signs take precedence over ultrasound findings which in turn take precedence over biochemical results (Figure 4.3). Flexibility is also key – never be afraid to change the planned treatment if the clinical picture alters.

Key points for clinical practice

- Assess symptoms first – moderate or severe pain indicates surgical intervention regardless of ultrasound findings or serum β-hCG results.
- The majority of ectopic pregnancies are visible on ultrasound.
- Laparoscopic total salpingectomy is the surgical treatment of choice for women with a healthy-looking contralateral tube.
- Systemic intramuscular methotrexate can be considered for selected women with β-hCG between 1500 and 5000 IU/L.
- Expectant management should be considered for selected women with β-hCG <1500 IU/L.
- The decision regarding the most appropriate treatment should be flexible and change in response to the clinical picture.

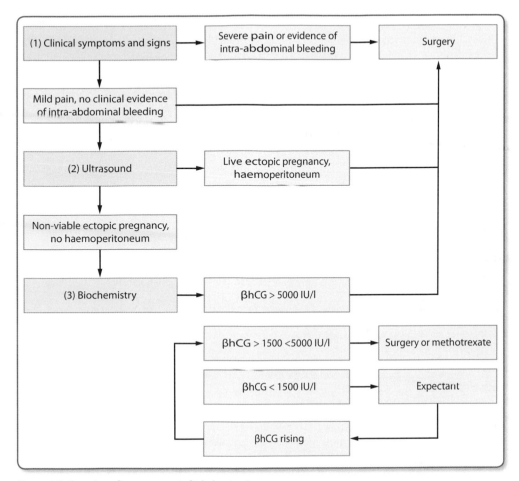

Figure 4.3 Overview of management of tubal ectopic pregnancy.

REFERENCES

1. Jurkovic D, Wilkinson H. Diagnosis and management of ectopic pregnancy. BMJ 2011; 342:3397.
2. Van Mello M, Mol F, Ankum W, et al. Ectopic pregnancy: how the diagnostic and therapeutic management has changed. Fertil Steril 2012; 98:1066–1073.
3. Cantwell R, Clutton-Brock T, Cooper G, et al. Saving mothers' lives: reviewing maternal deaths to make motherhood safer: 2006–2008. The eighth report of the confidential enquiries into maternal deaths in the United Kingdom. BJOG 2011; 118:1–203.
4. Casikar I, Reid S, Condous G. Ectopic pregnancy: ultrasound diagnosis in modern management. Clin Obstet Gynecol. 2012; 55:402–409.
5. Ankum VM, Mol BW, Van der Veen F, et al. Risk factors for ectopic pregnancy:a meta-analysis. Fertil Steril 1996; 65:1093–1099.
6. Jurkovic D, Mavrelos D. Catch me if you scan: ultrasound diagnosis of ectopic pregnancy. Ultrasound Obstet Gynecol 2007; 30:1–7.
7. Dutta RL, Economides DL. Patient acceptance of transvaginal sonography in the early pregnancy unit setting. Ultrasound Obstet Gynecol 2003; 22:503–507.
8. Condous G, Okaro E, Khalid A, et al. The accuracy of transvaginal ultrasonography for the diagnosis of ectopic pregnancy prior to surgery. Hum Reprod 2005; 20:1404–1409.

9. Kirk E, Papageorghiou AT, Condous G, et al. The diagnostic effectivness of an intital transvaginal scan in detecting ectopic pregnancy. Hum Reprod 2007; 22:2824–2828.
10. Ziel HK, Paulson RJ. Contralateral corpus luteum in ectopic pregnancy: what does it tell us about ovum pickup? Fertil Steril 2002; 77:850–851.
11. Kirk E. Ultrasound in the diagnosis of ectopic pregnancy. Clin Obstet Gynaecol 2012; 55:395–401.
12. Lavie O, Boldes R, Neuman M, et al. Ultrasonographic 'endometrial three-layer' pattern: a unique finding in ectopic pregnancy. J Clin Ultrasound 1996; 24:179–183.
13. Marks WM, Filly RA, Callen PW, et al. The decidual cast of ectopic pregnancy: a confusing ultrasonographic appearance. Radiology 1979; 133:451–454.
14. Sickler GK, Chen PC, Dubinsky TJ, et al. Free echogenic pelvic fluid: correlation with hemoperitoneum. J Ultrasound Med 1998; 17:431–435.
15. Popowski T, Huchon C, Toret-Labeeuw F, et al. Hemoperitoneum assessment in ectopic pregnancy. Int J Gynaecol Obstet 2012; 116:97–100.
16. Abrams BJ, Sukumvanich P, Seibel R, et al. Ultrasound for the detection of intraperitoneal fluid: The role of Trendelenburg positioning. Am J Emerg Med 1999; 17:117–120. .
17. Tulandi T, Hemmings R, Khalifa F. Rupture of ectopic pregnancy in women with low and declining serum beta-human chorionic gonadotropin concentrations. Fertil Steril 1991; 56:786–787.
18. Cordina M, Schramm-Gajraj K, Ross JA, et al. Introduction of a single visit protocol in the management of selected patients with pregnancy of unknown location: a prospective study. BJOG 2011; 118:693–697.
19. Newbatt E, Beckles Z, Ullman R, et al. Ectopic pregnancy and miscarriage: summary of NICE guidance. BMJ 2012; 345:e816.
20. Li TC, Tristram A, Hill AS, et al. A review of 254 ectopic pregnancies in a teaching hospital in the Trent Region, 1977–1990. Hum Reprod 1991; 6:1002–1007.
21. Kadar N. Early recourse to laparoscopy in the management of suspected ectopic pregnancy. Accuracy and morbidity. J Reprod Med 1990; 35:1153–1156.
22A. Mol F, Mol BW, Ankum WM, et al. Current evidence on surgery, systemic methotrexate and expectant management in the treatment of tubal ectopic pregnancy: a systematic review and meta-analysis. Hum Reprod Update 2008; 14:309–319.
22B. Mol F, van Mello NM, Strandell A, et al. Salpingotomy versus salpingectomy in women with tubal pregnancy (ESEP study): an open-label, multicentre, randomised controlled trial. Lancet 2014; Jan 31: pii: S0140-6736(14)60123-9. doi: 10.1016/S0140-6736(14)60123-9. [Epub ahead of print].
23. Chou LL, Huang MC. Recurrent ectopic pregnancy after ipsilateral segmental salpingectomy. Taiwan J Obstet Gynecol 2008; 47:203–205.
24. Stovall, TG Ling FW. Single-dose methotrexate: an expanded clinical trial. Am J Obstet Gynecol 1993; 168: 1759–1762; discussion 1762–1755.
25A. Lipscomb GH. Medical management of ectopic pregnancy. Clin Obstet Gynecol 2012; 55:424–432.
25B. Gervaise A, Masson L, de Tayrac R, et al. Reproductive outcome after methotrexate treatment of tubal pregnancies. Fertil Steril 2004; 82:304–308.
26. Nurmohamed L, Moretti ME, Schechter T, et al. Outcome following high-dose methotrexate in pregnancies misdiagnosed as ectopic. Am J Obstet Gynecol 2011; 205:533, e1–3.
27. Elson J, Tailor A, Banerjee S, et al. Expectant management of tubal ectopic pregnancy: prediction of successful outcome using decision tree analysis. Ultrasound Obstet Gynecol 2004; 23:552–556.
28. Craig LB, Khan S. Expectant management of ectopic pregnancy. Clin Obstet Gynecol 2012; 55:461–470.
29. Mavrelos D, Nicks H, Jamil A, et al. Efficacy and safety of a clinical protocol for expectant management of selected women diagnosed with a tubal ectopic pregnancy. Ultrasound Obstet Gynecol 2013; 42:102–107.
30. van Mello NM, Mol F, Verhoeve HR, et al. Methotrexate or expectant management in women with an ectopic pregnancy or pregnancy of unknown location and low serum hCG concentrations? A randomized comparison. Hum Reprod 2013; 28:60–67.

Chapter 5

Non-invasive prenatal diagnosis

David Lissauer, Stephanie Allen, Fiona Mackie, Mark D Kilby

INTRODUCTION

Prenatal diagnosis is a cornerstone of fetal medicine. The ability to obtain fetal genetic material upon which a diagnosis of problems such as fetal aneuploidy, or monogenic disorders can be made was traditionally reliant on invasive techniques, which carry an inherent risk of miscarriage. However, during the last 15 years, we have witnessed dramatic and rapid advances in this field, meaning that alternative non-invasive methods of obtaining and interrogating fetal genetic material are now a reality, yet the extremely fast progress means many clinicians have not been able to keep up with these advances. We therefore present an overview of the current state-of-the-art tests used to aid non-invasive prenatal diagnosis and non-invasive prenatal testing (NIPT) and the implications for clinical practice.

BACKGROUND

Historically, the search for fetal genetic material in the maternal circulation focussed on the isolation of intact fetal cells. Whilst fetal cells do circulate in the maternal circulation [1], they are very rare (approximately 1 cell per mL) [2] and technically challenging to isolate. Furthermore, it is now recognised that these fetal cells persist in the circulation beyond pregnancy [3] and cells from a previous pregnancy can even be detected many years later [4]. This persistence of fetal cells has potentially important consequences for maternal health [5] and also makes them a far less useful target from which to obtain fetal genetic material for the purposes of prenatal diagnosis.

David Lissauer PhD MBChB, Centre for Women's & Children's Health, University of Birmingham, Birmingham Women's Hospital, Birmingham, UK. Email: d.m.lissauer@bham.ac.uk (for correspondence)

Stephanie Allen PhD, Regional Genetics Laboratory, Birmingham Women's NHS Foundation Trust, Birmingham, UK

Fiona Mackie MBChB MRes, Centre for Women's & Children's Health, University of Birmingham, Birmingham Women's Hospital, Birmingham, UK.

Mark D Kilby DSc MD FRCOG, Centre for Women's & Children's Health, University of Birmingham, Birmingham Women's Hospital, Birmingham, UK.

A scientific breakthrough came in 1997 with the recognition that it was not necessary to detect intact fetal cells but that maternal plasma contained within it fetal cell-free DNA (cfDNA) [6]. It has been shown that this material mainly originates from fetal trophoblast [7] and consists of relatively short fragments of fetal DNA (143 base pairs on average) [8]. Recent work has demonstrated that cfDNA represents the whole of the fetal genome [9]. This has several crucial features that make it far more suitable for prenatal diagnosis than intact fetal cells. Firstly, cfDNA of fetal origin is present in relatively large quantities, representing up to 20% of the total maternal plasma DNA in later pregnancy [10]. It is also found from early in pregnancy, even from 4–5 weeks' gestation [10]. Furthermore, it is very rapidly cleared from the maternal circulation (with a half-life of 16 minutes) making it no longer detectable only hours after delivery [11]. The challenge is that fetal DNA still only represents a minority partner, mixed amongst the maternal DNA, and as such deciphering the fetal from the maternal signature is the major technical challenge. Early work focussed on the detection of genes known only to be present in the fetus. These included identifying genes on the Y chromosome from a male fetus, or other alleles present in the fetus alone, such as identifying a fetus which is rhesus positive in a rhesus negative mother. However, technological advances such as digital polymerase chain reactions (PCR) and massively parallel sequencing (MPS), which enable the far more precise enumeration of genes present in cfDNA, now mean that the far more difficult challenge of identifying a fetus with aneuploidy or even the sequencing of the entire fetal genome are now becoming a reality.

FETAL SEX DETERMINATION

One of the best established, and now widely available prenatal diagnostic tests on cfDNA, is for fetal sex determination. This is of considerable importance for carriers of X-linked genetic disorders, in which a male fetus is at particular risk, and early fetal sexing will enable appropriate counselling and an informed decision regarding whether a definitive diagnostic test is required. This test may also be important in a range of other clinical situations, in which knowledge of the gender is useful prior to 12 weeks, after which it can be determined by ultrasound, or in situations where the ultrasound findings are ambiguous and knowledge of the genetic sex is required [12].

The testing for fetal sex relies upon the detection of Y chromosome specific sequences in cfDNA present in maternal plasma. It is assumed that the presence of Y chromosome specific sequences is due to a male fetus. There have been two genes targeted for this test, the single copy SRY gene [2, 10, 13, 14] and the multicopy DYS14 [2, 14, 15]. A systematic review and meta-analysis of the diagnostic accuracy of this test which included 90 studies (9965 pregnancies) demonstrated that in the first trimester the test is 95.0% sensitive and 98.8% specific, with this increasing to 98.2% sensitivity and 99.5% specificity in the 2nd trimester [16]. This is consistent with other recent systematic reviews of the accuracy of the test [17]. The reason for this increasing accuracy at later gestations is the increase in the level of cfDNA in the maternal circulation [10, 15]. Before 5 [16] – 7 [17] weeks, the test is not as reliable due to the lower levels of fetal DNA increasing the risk of false negative results. The advent of methods to ensure adequate quantities of fetal DNA are present in the tested sample before testing is undertaken should reduce this false negative rate. In addition, accurate dating of the pregnancy is required to ensure the test is not undertaken too early, and ultrasound exclusion of a twin pregnancy or a 'vanishing twin' is also important as this is a potential source of a false positive result.

Non-invasive prenatal diagnosis of fetal sex is widely available in the UK and elsewhere. In the UK, the test is conducted through a number of specialised testing centres and has been shown to be reliable and practical in clinical practice [18]. Indeed, in women at high risk of sex-linked disorders fetal sex determination using cfDNA based approaches is now approved by the UK Genetic Testing Network and is integrated into the clinical pathway [19]. Its utility has been shown in a reduced need for subsequent invasive testing [20]. Economic analysis has demonstrated that for those conditions where patients would otherwise undergo invasive testing, the expense of the test is offset by the money saved avoiding invasive testing, making this cost neutral with potential benefits inherent in reducing the miscarriage risk [21].

RHESUS DETERMINATION

Incompatibility between the maternal and fetal rhesus D (RhD) blood group antigens is an important clinical problem. RhD status is determined by the presence of the RhD gene on chromosome 1, which is inherited in an autosomal dominant manner. Administration of anti-D to RhD negative mothers is normally conducted during pregnancy, to avoid maternal immunisation and the potential for haemolytic disease of the newborn in subsequent pregnancies. However, anti-D is a blood product, made from pooled plasma obtained from sensitised donors, with theoretical risks inherent in the use of blood products [22]. Furthermore, if given to all RhD negative mothers in a Caucasian population, 40% of these women will be receiving it unnecessarily as they are carrying a RhD negative fetus [23].

In RhD negative mothers the RhD gene is normally deleted and entirely absent, thus the detection of fetal RhD status is very similar to the detection of the Y chromosome in pregnancies affected by a male fetus. In RhD negative mothers, if following the interrogation of cfDNA there is evidence of the RhD gene this is assumed to have come from the fetus, and the fetus is therefore assumed to be RhD positive. If the examination reveals no RhD genes it is assumed the fetus is RhD negative. The clinical importance of this problem and the relative simplicity of detection meant that this was an early area for intense investigation [24, 25]. This early success has been followed by a raft of large studies that have very carefully defined the accuracy and clinical utility of these tests [26-30].

The technical approaches taken have also been similar to those utilised for fetal sex determination. Large scale studies have utilised quantitative real-time PCR because the technique is already in widespread use for other clinical tests, it is highly sensitive, robust and can be automated. Indeed high throughput systems using this approach have proven themselves to be effective [26]. However, alternative approaches such as mass spectrometric assays are also possible and may allow even higher throughput [31].

These large scale studies have demonstrated the very high degree of accuracy possible from these assays, with values ranging from an accuracy of 95.5-100% [23, 26, 28-30]. However, for this assay false positives are not the primary concern, as these women will simply receive an unnecessary dose of anti-D, as they would have done in routine practice prior to the use of cfDNA screening. The problem arises from false negative results, as these women would in error not be given anti-D and are at risk of becoming sensitised and future pregnancies could be put in jeopardy. Fortunately, these large scale studies have shown that the false negative rates are low and vary from 0-0.12% [23, 26, 28-30].

Significant improvements have been made since the early assays to reduce incorrect results. In particular, it is recognised that the rhesus system is more complex than was first assumed, and RhD pseudogenes occur, in which an individual will have an almost intact RhD gene but are serotypically RhD negative. This is particularly a feature in women of African descent (found in 66% of RhD negative black Africans) [32]. Other variants are also present such as RHD-CE-D which is also found in 22% of Rh negative African Americans [33]. In light of these observations it is recommended that additional PCR reactions are used, appropriate to the patients ethnicity, to enable variants common in that population to be excluded [34].

The demonstration of the accuracy of prenatal diagnosis of fetal RhD status from cfDNA from large studies has led to their widespread use in clinical practice. In pregnancies at high risk of rhesus disease, such as women already sensitised, knowledge of the fetal RhD status is crucial for management. For these women in settings where these tests are available they have virtually replaced invasive diagnostic procedures to determine fetal RhD status [35]. The area where uncertainty remains is regarding the implementation of such a testing strategy in a low-risk population, the practicalities of integrating such an effort into individual national health care and screening systems, and the cost benefit of such approaches. Indeed, routine testing at 25 weeks' gestation has already been successfully introduced into antenatal care in Denmark. [36]. In the UK recent guidance from the National Institute of Health and Clinical Excellence has recommended the exploration of routine antenatal fetal RhD typing [22].

ANEUPLOIDY DETECTION/NON-INVASIVE PRENATAL TESTING

The previously described uses of cfDNA analysis are technically less challenging because in both fetal sexing and RhD determination the DNA is being interrogated to find genes that would otherwise not be present in the mother. However, using cfDNA for the detection of fetal aneuploidy is more difficult as one is trying to establish a quantitative difference in the fetal contribution, amongst the cfDNA reservoir which also contains the maternal DNA as the majority (80%) [10, 37]. In these circumstances, such as a woman carrying a fetus with trisomy 21, one would expect the total amount of cfDNA originating from chromosome 21 would be higher than expected due to the additional fetal chromosome 21, however, this relative excess would be small because fetal DNA is only the minority of DNA present (Figure 5.1). A very precise technique for making these counts is therefore required to detect these small differences reliably and/or a technique is required to enrich the fetal cfDNA fraction.

Fetal cfDNA enrichment

A range of approaches have been attempted to selectively enrich the fetal cfDNA fraction. Firstly, there appears to be a physiological enrichment of cfDNA in pregnancies with Down's syndrome fetuses [38]. Artificial enrichment methods have included attempts to separate fetal and maternal DNA on the basis that fetal DNA fragments are typically smaller in size [39]. Chemical purification techniques have also been attempted [40], as well as immunoprecipitation methods based on differential DNA methylation (MeDIP-qPCR) [41, 42]. Further investigation is preparing such methods for clinical use in larger validation

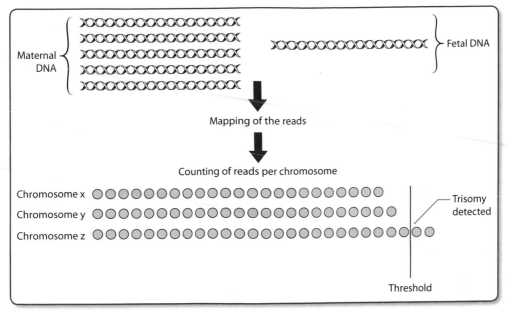

Figure 5.1 The use of massively parallel sequencing for the non-invasive prenatal detection of fetal chromosomal aneuploidy. (a) A mixture of maternal (blue) and fetal (red) DNA fragments are present in maternal plasma. The fetal DNA being up to 20% of the total cell free DNA. Sequencing technology is then used to sequence these DNA fragments. (b) These sequences are mapped to the human genome to identify the chromosome of origin of the sequences. (c) The number of sequences per chromosome are then counted. Various statistical techniques can then be employed to evaluate the number of reads from the chromosome of interest compared to the other chromosomes, and whether an excess of the chromosome is represented, as would be expected with fetal trisomy [67].

studies. Over time it will become clear which, if any, of these methods will become integrated as part of commonly used screening techniques or if advances in sequencing based approaches will supersede the need for enrichment.

Massively parallel sequencing

To accurately detect the small increases in the total amount of cfDNA from a particular chromosome that would be seen in fetal aneuploidy, extremely large numbers of the DNA fragments present in cfDNA must be counted. Massively parallel sequencing (MPS) approaches make this technically possible as they enable millions of DNA molecules to be analysed on a single run, with the ability to count and quantify the fragments and also through their sequence identify, by reference to the known human genome sequence, where on the genome the fragment originates [43].

Shotgun massively parallel sequencing approaches

The 'shotgun' approach involves a non-selective sequencing of all fragments. Though, inevitably most will not map to the chromosome or few chromosomes of interest. For example, chromosome 21 would represent <1.5% of sequenced fragments, so the number of counts required must be large enough to ensure sufficient fragments from chromosome 21 are identified to enable a difference between a euploid and a trisomic fetus to be seen [44].

This approach has been widely used and was the first MPS approach reported. Early studies by Fan [45] and Chiu [46] showed the feasibility of this method and a number of large scale validation studies have now been conducted **(Table 5.1)**. These studies have demonstrated that fetal aneuploidy detection can be conducted with very high sensitivity and specificity. NIPT utilising this approach is now available on a clinical basis through a number of companies worldwide.

However, challenges remain due to the cost and practicalities of such testing approaches, although sequencing costs are falling rapidly with time. In particular very large numbers of reads are required to ensure adequate test accuracy. Costs can be improved by running multiple samples at the same time. This is done by adding a 'bar-code' to each fragment that identifies which patient sample it corresponds to. The decision can therefore me made as to how many cases can be run at the same time, but this limits the number of reads per case. Chiu et al. demonstrated this as if the mean mappable sequence reads was reduced from 2.3 million (running two samples in parallel) to 0.3 million (running eight samples in parallel) there was a corresponding drop in test sensitivity from 100% to 79% for the detection of trisomy 21.

Targeted massively parallel sequencing approaches

In targeted MPS approaches, rather than sequencing across the whole genome techniques are used to target sequencing to chromosomes at risk of aneuploidy. This improves efficiency as less unused information is collected, and therefore also reduces sequencing costs. The relative merits and limitations of targeted versus shotgun approaches have been recently reviewed [44] and large scale trials using targeted approaches are summarised in **Table 5.1**. These demonstrate that this method has also been shown to perform well, with similar results across both approaches. Therefore, this approach is also offered clinically by a number of companies.

Methods utilised in the targeted approach include those that selectively amplify specific regions on chromosome 21 and 18, such as the digital analysis of selected regions (DANSR)

Table 5.1 Large validation studies using massively parallel sequencing based approaches for cfDNA screening for fetal trisomy [21]				
Study	Method	Detection rate (%)	False-positive rate (%)	No result* (%)
Chiu et al. [46]	Shotgun	86/86 (100)	3/146 (2.1)	11/764 (1.4)
Ehrich et al.	Shotgun	39/39 (100)	1/410 (0.2)	18/467 (3.9)
Palomaki et al.	Shotgun	209/212 (98.6)	3/1471 (0.2)	13/1686 (0.8)
Bianchi et al.[†]	Shotgun	90/90 (100)	6/410 (1.5)	16/532 (3.0)
Sparks et al. [47]	Targeted	36/36 (100)	1/123 (0.8)	8/338 (2.4)
Ashoor et al. [49]	Targeted	50/50 (100)	0/297 (0)	3/400 (0.8)
Norton et al. [50]	Targeted	81/81 (100)	3/2888 (0.1)	148/3228 (4.6)
Total		591/594 (99.5)	17/5745 (0.3)	217/7415 (2.9)

*Due to low fetal DNA levels or test failure.
† Results returned as unclassified have been counted as positive as these would be considered as 'high risk' and require further testing.

technique, which can reduce the number of reads to approximately 1 million required per sample. [47–50]. Other methods involve enrichment for single nucleotide polymorphism loci, which have also been shown to be effective in identifying the common trisomies [51].

Currently, whole genome MPS approaches are more extensively validated than targeted approaches for detection of aneuploidy. Although, targeted approaches are currently cheaper, they have the limitation of only being able to study the region being targeted by the assay. The on-going rapid reduction in the costs associated with sequencing, together with the potential for the detection of other aberrations such as aneuploidies of other chromosomes, and submicroscopic chromosomal aberrations, may mean that in the long term, the whole genome MPS approach becomes more attractive.

Intellectual property issues

The clinical translation of NIPT has largely been driven by industry and the huge commercial stakes involved. Technologies for isolation and genetic analysis of cfDNA have been patented by a small number of companies. These patents are currently the subject of on-going disputes and legal action between these companies that are yet to be resolved. How these patents will influence the clinical implementation of NIPT remains to be seen [52].

Clinical use of cfDNA testing for fetal aneuploidy

There are certain specific caveats to cfDNA testing for fetal aneuploidy in clinical practice that are important to consider:

These tests despite having demonstrated good test accuracy should not be considered fully diagnostic, and therefore do not currently offer a replacement for amniocentesis and CVS [53]. Women should therefore be advised that although false positive rates are low, they do occur and women with a positive test result should at this time therefore also be offered diagnostic invasive testing [53].

The reliance of cfDNA tests on the proportion of fetal cfDNA present in the plasma is an important consideration. The proportion of fetal DNA present increases with gestation [15] and to ensure adequate cfDNA is present these tests are normally advised to be used after 10 weeks' gestation [53]. Another situation where lower than expected amounts of cfDNA are found is in obese mothers [54].

Multiple pregnancies, lead to substantial additional complexity. Whilst it is technically possible to determine zygosity [55] and apply cfDNA testing to twin pregnancies this is not yet something recommended clinically as there is insufficient information to know how well the test performs in multiple pregnancies that are discordant for trisomy. Furthermore, false positive results could be obtained from a vanishing twin or empty gestation sac, and therefore ultrasound examination prior to cfDNA testing therefore remains important.

Placental mosaicism has been well described when fetal genetic material is obtained from CVS samples [56]. As cfDNA is predominantly of placental origin a similar phenomenon is seen to occur in a minority of cases, where there is discordance between the NIPT result and the fetal karyotype on confirmatory invasive procedures. Several examples of this have already been reported [57, 58]. Only with larger cohorts will the frequency of problems caused by this issue be revealed.

Whilst the accuracy of these tests has been demonstrated (**Table 5.1**) the widespread use of these tests in a low-risk population, or as part of routine testing remains to be determined. Currently international guidance reflects this opinion with the International

Society of Prenatal Diagnosis suggesting that cfDNA fetal aneuploidy testing may be offered to high-risk and not low-risk women [53]. The American Society of Obstetrics and Gynaecology similarly in an opinion statement in 2012 advised this can, with appropriate pre-test counselling, be used as a primary screening test in high-risk but not low-risk women [59]. Further work on the efficacy, cost effectiveness, practicality and acceptability of implementing NIPT as a primary or complementary part of national screening programmes for fetal aneuploidy is required.

SINGLE GENE DISORDERS

Our increasing knowledge of the underlying genetic basis of many diseases has led to an expansion in the demand for prenatal diagnosis of single gene disorders. Indeed, a recent audit of the UK Clinical Molecular Genetics Society demonstrated that prenatal diagnosis of over 150 different monogenic diseases was conducted over 1 year in the UK [60]. It would clearly be desirable if these conditions could be tested for non-invasively as most of these women are at a high-risk of having a child affected with a genetic disorder. However, to date, the money invested into development of non-invasive prenatal diagnosis (NIPD) for rare disorders is in stark contrast to the much larger sums invested into the development of NIPT for aneuploidy. Development of NIPD for single gene disorders also presents some difficult technical and practical challenges due to their diversity and rarity. Those that are technically more straightforward to detect are conditions which are X-linked where the diagnosis of fetal sex (as outlined above) can reduce the need for invasive testing. This was extended to autosomal dominant conditions that were either de novo mutations or paternally inherited. Examples of this include diagnosis of Huntington's disease [61] and achondroplasia [62].

Newer approaches mean that the challenge of non-invasive testing for autosomal recessive conditions is now also being tackled. This required technique to more accurately quantify the mutational load of the mixture of cfDNA containing both maternal and fetal material. Initial strategies were to exclude paternally inherited alleles, because if one could exclude the paternal allele being inherited then the fetus would at most be a carrier, and therefore invasive testing could be excluded. This has been done successfully with a range of techniques for disorders such as β-thalassemia [63] and cystic fibrosis [64]. In autosomal recessive conditions where both parents carry identical mutations, the paternally and maternally inherited alleles cannot be distinguished and novel techniques such as 'relative mutation dosage' (RMD) are required. This works on the principle that if the woman was heterozygous and the fetus is also heterozygous there will be 'allelic balance' between the diseased and normal alleles. However, if the fetus is homozygous for either the diseased or normal allele than one or other will be over-represented. This can be achieved using the technology of digital PCR, which enables a more precise enumeration of DNA copy number. The principle behind digital PCR is that the template DNA is diluted until there is on average less than one copy per reaction. Many hundreds of individual PCR reactions are then carried out, with the number of positive reactions corresponding to the number of wells that contained a copy of the DNA, and therefore precise counting of the starting copy number is possible [65] There are a number of platforms that make this approach possible. In addition, the development on bench top sequencing platforms may provide an alternative flexible approach to NIPD for single gene disorders. The use of digital PCR and other technologies in diagnosis of single gene disorders has been recently reviewed, providing more details on the specific platforms [66].

ETHICAL CONSIDERATIONS

The potential for non-invasive testing to reduce the need for invasive testing, and consequently decrease the inherent risk of miscarriage that this poses to normal fetuses is an important opportunity of this technology, which may alleviate some of the current ethical problems associated with current screening and testing approaches. However, this new technology does also bring new ethical challenges. The risks of invasive testing mean that considerable thought and counselling is undertaken prior to the procedure. The simplicity of non-invasive diagnosis based on a maternal peripheral blood sample early in pregnancy means there may be an increased risk that adequate counselling will not be undertaken.

Furthermore, with the increasing sophistication of the technology and the expanding possibilities offered by sequencing technology it may be possible to screen for multiple diseases simultaneously, and this poses difficulties in providing appropriate informed consent for all the potential disorders that may be being investigated. There are also the possibilities of screening not only for serious diseases but for other genetic traits such as those associated with increased risks of adult cancer or associations with other late onset disorders, and decisions must be made by society as well as individuals about where the limits of acceptable screening lie.

Additional concerns also centre around nonmedical uses of this technology. Particularly, the relative ease of early fetal sexing which could be abused for reasons of gender preference or the potential for paternity testing to be conducted prenatally.

CONCLUSION

The discovery of cfDNA in the maternal circulation has opened up the possibility to interrogate the fetal genome prenatally. This combined with the on-going revolution in molecular genetics, including huge advances in sequencing technology, now also enables this fetal material to be interrogated in detail. It is predicted that within the next decade the problems of cost and throughput currently being tackled will be solved and prenatal diagnosis will become predominantly a non-invasive process.

Key points for clinical practice

- Cell free DNA can be isolated from maternal plasma. This contains fetal genetic material, which allows the non-invasive interrogation of the fetal genome.

- Fetal rhesus status and fetal sex can be non-invasively determined by well-validated assays. These tests are a useful tool in the management of high-risk women, where available, and can be done from the 1st trimester. Ultrasound is required to date the pregnancy and rule out multiple gestation prior to testing.

- Non-invasive prenatal testing for fetal aneuploidy has also been well-validated in high-risk groups and may be offered to these women, with special counselling. However, this technology remains costly and the best way that this should be integrated into current screening approaches remains to be determined. Currently guidelines do not recommend its use in low-risk women.

- Information that should be provided to pregnant women wanting to undergo cfDNA testing for fetal aneuploidy (Guidance from the position statement of the Board of the International Society for Prenatal Diagnosis [53]) includes detailed counselling on the benefits and limitations of the tests, and notification that these tests are still under clinical development. They must be informed that:

  a. Currently available tests mostly focus on detection of fetal trisomies 21, 18 and 13.

  b. Detection rates are high, but testing does not detect all cases of these trisomies.

  c. False positive results do occur, albeit at a low rate, therefore, women with positive results should be offered confirmatory chromosome analysis by invasive testing.

  d. For some women cfDNA testing may not be informative and they may then need to consider a screening test and/or invasive testing. In particular women with an increased body mass index are at risk of test failure or an inconclusive result. For late gestational age women this may lead to delays and insufficient time for a repeat screening test and/or invasive test.

REFERENCES

1. Lo YM, Lo ES, Watson N, et al. Two-way cell traffic between mother and fetus: biologic and clinical implications. Blood 1996; 88:4390–4395.
2. Zhong XY, Holzgreve W, Hahn S. Direct quantification of fetal cells in maternal blood by real-time PCR 50. Prenat Diagn 2006; 26:850–854.
3. Bianchi DW, Zickwolf GK, Weil GJ, et al. Male fetal progenitor cells persist in maternal blood for as long as 27 years postpartum. Proc Natl Acad Sci USA 1996; 93:705–708.
4. Lissauer DM, Piper KP, Moss PA, et al. Fetal microchimerism: the cellular and immunological legacy of pregnancy. Expert Rev Mol Med 2009; 11:e33.
5. Lissauer D, Piper KP, Moss PA, et al. Persistence of fetal cells in the mother: friend or foe? BJOG 2007; 114:1321–1325.
6. Lo YM, Corbetta N, Chamberlain PF, et al. Presence of fetal DNA in maternal plasma and serum. Lancet 1997; 350:485–487.
7. Alberry M, Maddocks D, Jones M, et al. Free fetal DNA in maternal plasma in anembryonic pregnancies: confirmation that the origin is the trophoblast. Prenat Diagn 2007; 27:415–418.
8. Lo YM, Chan KC, Sun H, et al. Maternal plasma DNA sequencing reveals the genome-wide genetic and mutational profile of the fetus. Sci Transl Med 2010; 2:61ra91.
9. Fan HC, Gu W, Wang J, et al. Non-invasive prenatal measurement of the fetal genome. Nature 2012; 487:320–324.
10. Lo YM, Tein MS, Lau TK, et al. Quantitative analysis of fetal DNA in maternal plasma and serum: implications for noninvasive prenatal diagnosis 18. Am J Hum Genet 1998; 62:768–775.
11. Lo YM, Zhang J, Leung TN, et al. Rapid clearance of fetal DNA from maternal plasma. Am J Hum Genet 1999:64:218–224.
12. Finning KM, Chitty LS. Non-invasive fetal sex determination: impact on clinical practice. Semin Fetal Neonatal Med 2008; 13:69–75.
13. Lo YM, Lau TK, Chan LY, Leung TN, et al. Quantitative analysis of the bidirectional fetomaternal transfer of nucleated cells and plasma DNA 48. Clin Chem 2000; 46:1301–1309.
14. Zimmermann B, El-Sheikhah A, Nicolaides K, et al. Optimized real-time quantitative PCR measurement of male fetal DNA in maternal plasma 3. Clin Chem 2005; 51:1598–1604.
15. Lissauer D, Piper K, Goodyear O, et al. Fetal-specific CD8+ cytotoxic T cell responses develop during normal human pregnancy and exhibit broad functional capacity. J Immunol 2012; 189:1072–1080.
16. Wright CF, Wei Y, Higgins JP, et al. Non-invasive prenatal diagnostic test accuracy for fetal sex using cell-free DNA a review and meta-analysis. BMC Res Notes 2012; 5: 476.
17. Devaney SA, Palomaki GE, Scott JA, et al. Noninvasive fetal sex determination using cell-free fetal DNA: a systematic review and meta-analysis. JAMA 2011; 306:627–636.

18. Hill M, Lewis C, Jenkins L, et al. Implementing noninvasive prenatal fetal sex determination using cell-free fetal DNA in the United Kingdom. Expert Opin Biol Ther. 2012; 12:s119–126.
19. UK Genetic Testing Network. Best practice guidelines for non-invasive prenatal diagnosis to determine fetal sex for known carriers of congenital adrenal hyperplasia (CAH), 2010. London: UK Genetic Testing Network, 2010.
20. Hill M, Finning K, Martin P, et al. Non-invasive prenatal determination of fetal sex: translating research into clinical practice. Clin Genet 2011; 80:68–75.
21. Hill M, Taffinder S, Chitty LS, et al. Incremental cost of non-invasive prenatal diagnosis versus invasive prenatal diagnosis of fetal sex in England. Prenat Diagn 2011; 31:267–273.
22. National Institute for Clinical Excellence (NICE). Routine antenatal anti-D prophylaxis for women who are rhesus D negative. Review of NICE technology appraisal guidance 41. London: NICE, 2008.
23. Van der Schoot CE, Soussan AA, Koelewijn J, et al. Non-invasive antenatal RhD typing. Transfus Clin Biol 2006; 13:53–57.
24. Lo YM, Hjelm NM, Fidler C, et al. Prenatal diagnosis of fetal RhD status by molecular analysis of maternal plasma. N Engl J Med 1998; 339: 1734–1738.
25. Faas BH, Beuling EA, Christiaens GC, et al. Detection of fetal RhD-specific sequences in maternal plasma. Lancet 1998; 352:1196.
26. Finning K, Martin P, Summers J, et al. Effect of high throughput RhD typing of fetal DNA in maternal plasma on use of anti-RhD immunoglobulin in RhD negative pregnant women: prospective feasibility study. BMJ 2008; 336:816–818.
27. Minon JM, Gerard C, Senterre JM, et al. Routine fetal RhD genotyping with maternal plasma: a 4-year experience in Belgium. Transfusion 2008; 48:373–381.
28. Rouillac-Le Sciellour C, Sérazin V, Brossard Y, et al. Noninvasive fetal RhD genotyping from maternal plasma. Use of a new developed Free DNA Fetal Kit RhD. Transfus Clin Biol 2007; 14:572–577.
29. Costa, JM, Giovangrandi Y, Ernault P, et al. Fetal RhD genotyping in maternal serum during the first trimester of pregnancy. Br J Haematol 2002; 119:255–260.
30. Gautier E, Benachi A, Giovangrandi Y, et al. Fetal RhD genotyping by maternal serum analysis: a 2-year experience. Am J Obstet Gynecol 2005; 192:666–669.
31. Bombard, AT, Akolekar R, Farkas DH, et al. Fetal RhD genotype detection from circulating cell-free fetal DNA in maternal plasma in non-sensitized RhD negative women. Prenat Diagn 2011; 31:802–808.
32. Singleton BK, Green CA, Avent ND, et al. The presence of an RhD pseudogene containing a 37 base pair duplication and a nonsense mutation in africans with the RhD-negative blood group phenotype. Blood 2000; 95:12–18.
33. Van der Schoot CE, Hahn S, Chitty LS. Non-invasive prenatal diagnosis and determination of fetal Rh status. Semin Fetal Neonatal Med 2008; 13:63–68.
34. Wright CF, Burton H. The use of cell-free fetal nucleic acids in maternal blood for non-invasive prenatal diagnosis. Hum Reprod Update 2009; 15:139–151.
35. Daniels G, Finning K, Martin P, et al. Fetal blood group genotyping: present and future. Ann NY Acad Sci. 2006; 1075:88–95.
36. Clausen FB, Christiansen M, Steffensen R, et al. Report of the first nationally implemented clinical routine screening for fetal RhD in D-pregnant women to ascertain the requirement for antenatal RhD prophylaxis. Transfusion, 2012; 52:752–758.
37. Lun FM, Chiu RW, Allen Chan KC, et al. Microfluidics digital PCR reveals a higher than expected fraction of fetal DNA in maternal plasma. Clin Chem. 2008; 54:1664–1672.
38. Lo YM, Lau TK, Zhang J, et al. Increased fetal DNA concentrations in the plasma of pregnant women carrying fetuses with trisomy 21. Clin Chem. 1999; 45:1747–1751.
39. Li Y, Zimmermann B, Rusterholz C, et al. Size separation of circulatory DNA in maternal plasma permits ready detection of fetal DNA polymorphisms. Clin Chem, 2004; 50:1002–1011.
40. Dhallan R, Au WC, Mattagajasingh S, et al. Methods to increase the percentage of free fetal DNA recovered from the maternal circulation. JAMA, 2004; 291:1114–1119.
41. Papageorgiou EA, Fiegler H, Rakyan V, et al. Sites of differential DNA methylation between placenta and peripheral blood: molecular markers for noninvasive prenatal diagnosis of aneuploidies. Am J Pathol 2009; 174:1609–1618.
42. Kyriakou S, Kypri E, Spyrou C, et al. Variability of ffDNA in maternal plasma does not prevent correct classification of trisomy 21 using MeDIP-qPCR methodology. Prenat Diagn 2013; 33:650–655.
43. Metzker ML. Sequencing technologies − the next generation. Nat Rev Genet 2010; 11:31–46.

44. Boon EM, Faas BH. Benefits and limitations of whole genome versus targeted approaches for noninvasive prenatal testing for fetal aneuploidies. Prenat Diagn 2013; 33:563–568.
45. Fan HC, Blumenfeld YJ, Chitkara U, et al. Noninvasive diagnosis of fetal aneuploidy by shotgun sequencing DNA from maternal blood. Proc Natl Acad Sci USA 2008; 105:16266–16271.
46. Chiu RW, Chan KC, Gao Y, et al. Noninvasive prenatal diagnosis of fetal chromosomal aneuploidy by massively parallel genomic sequencing of DNA in maternal plasma. Proc Natl Acad Sci USA 2008; 105:20458–20463.
47. Sparks AB, Struble CA, Wang ET, et al. Noninvasive prenatal detection and selective analysis of cell-free DNA obtained from maternal blood: evaluation for trisomy 21 and trisomy 18. Am J Obstet Gynecol 2012; 206:319 e1–9.
48. Sparks AB, Wang ET, Struble CA, et al. Selective analysis of cell-free DNA in maternal blood for evaluation of fetal trisomy. Prenat Diagn 2012; 32:3–9.
49. Ashoor G, Syngelaki A, Wagner M, et al. Chromosome-selective sequencing of maternal plasma cell-free DNA for first-trimester detection of trisomy 21 and trisomy 18. Am J Obstet Gynecol. 2012; 206:322 e1–5.
50. Norton ME, Brar H, Weiss J, et al. Non-invasive chromosomal evaluation (NICE) study: results of a multicenter prospective cohort study for detection of fetal trisomy 21 and trisomy 18. Am J Obstet Gynecol 2012; 207:137 e1–8.
51. Zimmermann B, Hill M, Gemelos G, et al. Noninvasive prenatal aneuploidy testing of chromosomes 13, 18, 21, X, and Y, using targeted sequencing of polymorphic loci. Prenat Diagn 2012; 32:1233–1241.
52. Agarwal A, Sayres LC, Cho MK, et al. Commercial landscape of noninvasive prenatal testing in the United States. Prenat Diagn 2013; 33:521–531.
53. Benn P, Borell A, Chiu R, et al. Position statement from the Aneuploidy Screening Committee on behalf of the Board of the International Society for Prenatal Diagnosis. Prenat Diagn 2013; 33:622–629.
54. Ashoor G, Syngelaki A, Poon LC, et al. Fetal fraction in maternal plasma cell-free DNA at 11–13 weeks' gestation: relation to maternal and fetal characteristics. Ultrasound Obstet Gynecol 2013; 41:26–32.
55. Qu JZ, Leung TY, Jiang P, et al. Noninvasive prenatal determination of twin zygosity by maternal plasma DNA analysis. Clin Chem 2013; 59:427–435.
56. Kalousek DK, Vekemans M. Confined placental mosaicism. J Med Genet 1996; 33:529–533.
57. Pan M, Li FT, Li Y, et al. Discordant results between fetal karyotyping and non-invasive prenatal testing by maternal plasma sequencing in a case of uniparental disomy 21 due to trisomic rescue. Prenat Diagn 2013; 33:598–601.
58. Lau TK, Jiang FM, Stevenson RJ, et al. Secondary findings from non-invasive prenatal testing for common fetal aneuploidies by whole genome sequencing as a clinical service. Prenat Diagn 2013; 33:602–608.
59. ACOG Committee Opinion No. 545: Non-invasive prenatal testing for fetal aneuploidy. Obstet Gynecol 2012; 120:1532–1534.
60. Clinical Molecular Genetics Society Audit of Data 2011–2012. London: Clinical Molecular Genetics Society, 2012. http://www.cmgs.org/CMGS audit/2012 audit/CMGSAudit11_12_FINAL.pdf.
61. Gonzalez-Gonzalez MC, Trujillo MJ, Rodríguez de Alba M. Huntington disease-unaffected fetus diagnosed from maternal plasma using QF-PCR. Prenat Diagn 2003; 23:232–234.
62. Saito H, Sekizawa A, Morimoto T, et al. Prenatal DNA diagnosis of a single-gene disorder from maternal plasma. Lancet 2000; 356:1170.
63. Galbiati S, Brisci A, Lalatta F, et al. Full COLD-PCR protocol for non-invasive prenatal diagnosis of genetic diseases. Clin Chem 2011; 57:136–138.
64. González-González MC, García-Hoyos M, Trujillo MJ, et al. Prenatal detection of a cystic fibrosis mutation in fetal DNA from maternal plasma. Prenat Diagn 2002; 22:946–948.
65. Vogelstein B, Kinzler KW. Digital PCR. Proc Natl Acad Sci USA 1999; 96:9236–9241.
66. Lench N, Barrett A, Fielding S, et al. The clinical implementation of non-invasive prenatal diagnosis for single-gene disorders: challenges and progress made. Prenat Diagn 2013; 33:555–562.
67. Nepomnyashchaya YN, Artemov AV, Roumiantsev SA, et al. Non-invasive prenatal diagnostics of aneuploidy using next-generation DNA sequencing technologies, and clinical considerations. Clin Chem Lab Med 2013; 51:1141–1154.
68. Ehrich M, Deciu C, Zwiefelhofer T, et al. Noninvasive detection of fetal trisomy 21 by sequencing of DNA in maternal blood: a study in a clinical setting Am J Obstet Gynecol 2011; 204:205.e1-11.
69. Palomaki GE, Kloza E, Lambert-Messerlian GM, et al. DNA sequencing of maternal plasma to detect Down syndrome: An international clinical validation study. Genet Med 2011; 13:913-920.
70. Bianchi DW, Platt LD, Goldberg JD, et al. Genome-wide fetal aneuploidy detection by maternal plasma DNA sequencing. Obstet Gynecol 2012; 113:890-901.

Chapter 6

Prevention of stillbirth

Alexander Heazell

INTRODUCTION

Stillbirth, defined by the World Health Organisation as fetal death after 28 weeks' gestation, accounts for an estimated 2.65 million deaths worldwide each year [1]. The majority of these deaths occur in low-or middle-income countries, with only 2% estimated to occur in high-income countries; in 2009, 76.2% of stillbirths occurred in South Asia and Sub-Saharan Africa. There are huge variations in the stillbirth rate between low-income and high-income settings, with the highest reported rates of stillbirth in Nigeria (41.9 per 1,000 births) and Pakistan (46.1 per 1,000 births) contrasting markedly with Finland (2.0 per 1,000 births), which has one of the lowest rates [1]. The causes of stillbirth differ between low-and high-income settings, and even within countries; the stillbirth rate in rural northern Nigeria is significantly greater than urban teaching hospitals in southern Nigeria [2]. In low-income settings (e.g. South Asia and Sub-Saharan Africa), up to 50% of stillbirths occur intrapartum, and relate to the absence of skilled birth-attendants and low access to caesarean section, factors which are particularly important in rural areas [2]. Thus, interventions to reduce stillbirth need to be targeted and relevant to individual populations.

The variance in stillbirth rates is not confined to the stark contrast between high-income countries and low-income countries. A detailed analysis of stillbirth rates (after 28 weeks' gestation) in 14 high-income settings demonstrated that the United Kingdom (UK) has the highest stillbirth rate of those analysed at 3.8 per 1,000 births **(Figure 6.1)** [3]. The overall stillbirth rate in high-income countries fell by 20.3% between 1990 and 2009. However, this reduction was not uniform across the high-income countries studied; Norway and the Netherlands reported a fall of 50% and 40% respectively. Norway reported a stillbirth rate after 28 weeks' gestation of 2.2 per 1,000 births in 2009, 42% lower than that of the UK. In the UK, where stillbirth is defined as an infant born with no signs of life after 24 completed weeks' gestation, there has been little or no reduction in stillbirth rates over the same time period **(Figure 6.1B)**. Variation in population characteristics, health behaviours and health care provision between high-income countries may explain some of the diverging data. However, the magnitude of the observed variation in stillbirth rates between countries and the difference in rates of reduction of stillbirth suggest that a decrease in stillbirth rates in the UK remains achievable. This contention is further supported by data from 2008, which showed that 84% of stillborn infants in the UK were >500 g and had no congenital abnormality, indicating that with appropriate intervention these infants may have survived

Alexander Heazell MBChB(Hons) PhD MRCOG, Maternal and Fetal Health Research Centre, University of Manchester, St Mary's Hospital, Manchester, UK. Email: alexander.heazell@manchester.ac.uk (for correspondence)

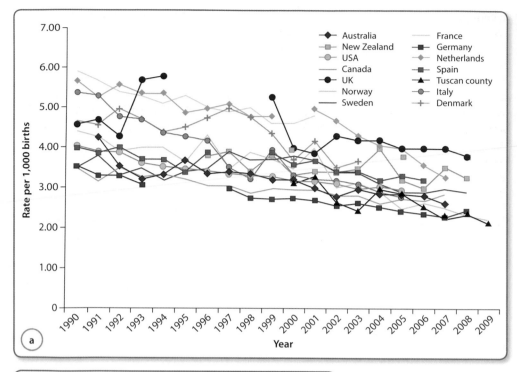

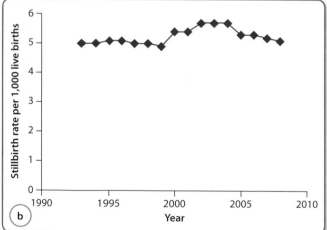

Figure 6.1A and B (a) Stillbirth rates from fourteen high-income settings. The UK has the highest rate of late-stillbirths (3.8 per 1,000 births). (b) The UK stillbirth rate (≥24 weeks) from 1994 to 2008 demonstrating very little change for almost two decades. With permission from Flenady et al, 2011.

[4]. Furthermore, 34% of stillborn infants were born after 37 weeks' gestation when delivery could have prevented stillbirth with minimal impact on short-term neonatal complications or longer-term outcome [4]. Therefore, at the simplest level a reduction in stillbirths is likely to be achievable in the UK, by inducing labour, an intervention that is associated with minimal maternal or fetal risks at term [5].

    A reduction in stillbirth rates is not only achievable but highly desirable. Stillbirth has a profound impact on parents' physical and mental health, social relationships within and outside the extended family and on employment [6]. The impact on physical health extends into subsequent pregnancies which are at a 2–10-fold increased risk of stillbirth depending upon the cause of the initial stillbirth. Rates of preterm birth and fetal growth restriction are also increased in women who have a history of stillbirth [7, 8]. The societal impact of the far-reaching consequences of stillbirth is difficult to quantify in a formal analysis. Notwithstanding this challenge, conservative estimates of the health care after stillbirth ranged from $1,450 in a 2002 study from the United States to £1,804 in a 2010 study from the UK [9A]. Guidelines from the National Institute of Health and Clinical Excellence (NICE) estimate the number of quality-adjusted life years (QALYs) lost from stillbirth is 25 based upon an approximate lifetime QALYs from 75 years lived in perfect health discounted at 3.5% per annum [9B]. However, this economic model this takes no account of QALYs lost from parents [10]. Litigation costs from stillbirth in the UK were reported by Mead's review of 100 stillbirth claims filed between 2003 and 2007; a total of £1,761,638 was paid in damages for 62 cases, averaging £28,413 per successful claim [11].

Thus, there are strong medical, economical and societal arguments to reduce the UK stillbirth rate. The International Stillbirth Alliance has called on countries with a stillbirth rate greater than 5 per 1,000 births to reduce rates by 50% by 2020, and those with a stillbirth rate lower than 5 per 1,000 to eliminate all preventable stillbirths and reduce inequalities resulting in stillbirth [12]. This manuscript will consider stillbirth prevention in the UK context, in the light of the earlier proposal that interventions to reduce the stillbirth rate should be targeted and relevant to individual populations.

THE CHALLENGE OF STILLBIRTH PREVENTION

Prevention of stillbirth is a challenge to public health and maternity care services in the UK. It requires a multidisciplinary approach with insight from basic scientists, epidemiologists, midwives, obstetricians, public health services, clinical trialists, parents and service users. A simplified pathway focussing on the prevention of stillbirth is shown in **Figure 6.2**. The most direct means of affecting stillbirth is shown in the highlighted boxes (in green), where understanding of the causes of and risk factors for stillbirth leads to the

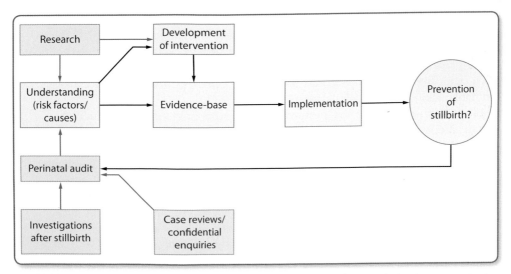

Figure 6.2 Hypothetical model for stillbirth prevention involving perinatal audit, research, development, evaluation and implementation of interventions.

development of evidence-based interventions which can then be implemented. The impact of developments in care can be assessed through perinatal audit, which then goes on to improve understanding of the cause of stillbirth in a cycle of improvement. Understanding the underlying causes of stillbirth is informed by research to better understand the aetiology and pathophysiology of stillbirth and epidemiological studies to identify relevant risk factors. Information regarding the causes of stillbirth in individual populations, which may be local, regional and national, can also be provided by perinatal audit. The perinatal audit process usually relies on information gathered from individual cases of stillbirth and in some cases, confidential inquiries or case reviews. Due to their fundamental importance to the prevention of stillbirth, the role of research and perinatal audit will be considered.

The role of perinatal audit

Perinatal audit is defined as 'the systematic critical analysis of the quality of perinatal care, including the procedures used for diagnosis and treatment, the use of resources and the resultant outcome and quality of life for women and their babies' [13]. At a basic level, perinatal audit provides information about the number of stillbirths and relevant demographic information, such as gestation at death/delivery, number of fetuses, maternal age, deprivation, etc. A more detailed data collection attempts to review the case and care provided and wherever possible determine the cause of the stillbirth. Perinatal audit is a dynamic process, where a better understanding of the causes of stillbirth, populations at increased risk and problems with delivery of care, allows recommendations to be developed and implemented, which are then re-evaluated. Although there have not been any randomised controlled trials of perinatal audit, there is evidence from 'before and after' case-control studies in high-income countries showing a substantial reduction in stillbirth rates following the introduction of perinatal audit. A fall in antenatal and neonatal deaths in northern Norway from 13.8 per 1,000 births to 7.7 per 1,000 births was noted following the introduction of audit [14]. In 1958 at the time of introduction of perinatal audit in the UK, the perinatal mortality rate was 21.5 per 1,000 births and this figure had fallen to 7.5 per 1,000 by 2008 [4, 15]. Whilst the observed falls in perinatal mortality can be attributed to many developments in maternity care, these improvements have undoubtedly been informed by data and analysis provided by published perinatal audits. In the UK, the co-ordination of perinatal audit is now the responsibility of the 'Mothers and babies: reducing risk through audits and confidential enquiries (MBRRACE) collaboration' (https://www.npeu.ox.ac.uk/mbrrace-uk) who have an online data collection for all perinatal deaths (with infant and maternal deaths) from 1st January 2013.

In addition to data collection, detailed perinatal audit makes use of confidential enquiry methodology where anonymised case notes are used to review the narrative of the case by a multidisciplinary team of experts. This extends the utility of the audit process from recording demographic data and determining the cause of death to evaluating the quality of care provided, recording whether the care is optimal or suboptimal, and if there was evidence of suboptimal care, whether this contributed to the stillbirth. Due to the intensive nature of this process, these reviews are usually confined to a specific group (e.g. intrapartum deaths) or geographical area. Studies from different high-income countries (Netherlands, Norway, UK) have found evidence of suboptimal care in 25–45% of cases [14, 16, 17]. Similar themes have been identified in all settings including failure to recognise high-risk status, failure to detect complications particularly fetal growth restriction (FGR), and failure to act. Other problems with care include poor communication between staff, women and their families. It is essential that these enquiries generate plans to address the problems identified. These investigations should be well-organised, ideally using a specific, measurable, acceptable and realistic, and time restricted (SMART) approach. Strategies to bring about change should be tailored to individual situations and appreciate barriers to their implementation [18].

The quality of data and tools used to interpret the information are essential to the success of perinatal audit, particularly in determining the cause of stillbirths. It is notable that even in regions or countries with developed structures for perinatal audit, including registration of deaths, protocols for investigation and classification of stillbirths, a complete dataset of demographic data and investigations was not available in a significant proportion of cases [19, 20]. Incomplete data limits the value of perinatal audit by restricting the ability to determine the cause of stillbirth, which is analogous to attempting to solve a crime with a significant proportion of the evidence missing. A detailed review of 1025 deaths in the Netherlands found the four investigations most likely to find useful or new information, or confirm the suspected cause of stillbirth were postmortem (autopsy), histopathological examination of the placenta, chromosomal analysis and a Kleihauer test, which detected abnormalities in 51.5%, 89.2%, 11.9%, and 11.9% of cases respectively [20]. Other tests also provide information, but are recommended for use in specific clinical situations guided by maternal history and clinical examination of the mother and baby [21]. In addition to the data collected, the classification system applied to stillbirths affects the proportion of stillbirths classified as unexplained. Older classification systems including modified Aberdeen and Wigglesworth, record higher levels of unexplained stillbirths (47.4%) compared to modern classification systems including ReCoDe (Relevant Conditions at Death) and Tulip which report 14.2% and 16.2% unexplained stillbirths in the same patient group [22]. Ideally, perinatal audit will make use of the maximum data available to determine factors which may be causative or associated with stillbirth in combination with a modern classification system. The combination of this information and that from detailed case reviews will facilitate the development and implementation of interventions to prevent stillbirth.

The role of research

Despite its impact, stillbirth is under-researched when compared to other pregnancy complications, e.g. a PubMed search using stillbirth (on 10/08/13) retrieves 5,738 hits in comparison to 17,822 for fetal growth restriction, 19,421 for preterm labour and 28,771 for pre-eclampsia. Research has an essential role to play in stillbirth prevention. Firstly, epidemiological studies provide information regarding risk factors for stillbirth; with regard to prevention, the most important of these are those amenable to modification. Risk factors identified by studies include social factors such as inequality with higher stillbirth rates in minority populations, indigenous populations, socially and economically deprived groups and women with low educational attainment. Other risk factors relating to maternal characteristics include maternal obesity, advanced maternal age and cigarette smoking. Medical factors and those relating to pregnancy include the increased stillbirth rate in prolonged pregnancy (>41 weeks), multiple pregnancy, pre-existing diabetes mellitus and hypertensive disorders of pregnancy [3]. Recently, the Auckland stillbirth study, a case-control study of 155 women with stillbirths and 310 gestational-age matched controls identified maternal sleep position as a novel risk factor associated with late stillbirth, with women who reported a right-sided sleep position on the night before the stillbirth at a 2.5-fold increased risk compared to left-sided sleeping [23]. Further evidence is needed before the relationship between sleep position and stillbirth can be confirmed. In addition, this study also established the association between previously reported risk factors including reduced fetal movements and cigarette smoking.

Secondly, research is required to improve understanding of the pathophysiology of stillbirth. This has two important aims pertinent to stillbirth prevention. The first is to provide information to understand how risk factors translate into stillbirth, e.g. diabetes is a recognised risk factor for stillbirth, but the reason for death and why two babies in similar clinical cases have different outcomes is unknown. The second is to facilitate the development of relevant investigations and therapies to identify fetuses at greatest risk of stillbirth and then intervene to prevent it. This requires high-quality translational research to generate research questions from the clinical environment to be tested and investigated using appropriate basic science techniques; the information from which informs clinical studies.

The International Stillbirth Alliance carried out a child health and nutrition research initiative (CHNRI) exercise in 2011 to determine the key research priorities relating to discovery, epidemiology and development, and delivery of care in high-income countries [3]. The top three priorities with regard to epidemiological research were to: (i) determine factors contributing to the excess in stillbirth rates in minority populations, (ii) understand which maternal lifestyle consumptions (e.g. caffeine, alcohol, substance misuse) are associated with stillbirth and their relation with other relevant disorders and causes of stillbirth, and (iii) identify the optimum investigation protocol for stillbirth to identify causes and relevant conditions in terms of yield, utility and costs. The top three ranked discovery priorities were: (i) the effects of periconceptual environment, including nutrition and micronutrient status, on embryonic development, (ii) development of repositories of well-phenotyped human samples from stillbirths or other related conditions and matched controls, and (iii) characterising the fetal response to an adverse intrauterine environment to develop improved means of clinical assessment of fetal wellbeing.

Thirdly, research into stillbirth prevention requires studies to evaluate changes in care to generate an evidence base, which can be evaluated and incorporated into guidelines for care. A systematic-review assessing the evidence-base for the prevention of stillbirths found a dearth of evidence for the direct impact of screening procedures and interventions on the incidence of stillbirth [24]. Much of the available evidence relies on observational studies such as 'before and after' studies rather than randomised controlled studies. This systematic review highlighted the need for large, adequately controlled trials to demonstrate the impact of interventions to reduce stillbirths. However, because of the relative infrequency of stillbirth, this requires development of more sophisticated methodology for comparative trials to develop feasible studies. For example, in a traditional randomised controlled trial to evaluate an intervention in women reporting reduced fetal movements (RFM), where the risk of stillbirth is three-times greater than the background risk [25], 146,945 patients per arm would be required to detect a 20% reduction in stillbirths after 36 weeks' gestation. An alternative approach using randomisation after testing, which assumes that women with a positive test are at a 4-fold increased risk of poor perinatal outcome, would require 5,568 participants in each arm to demonstrate a 20% decrease in the stillbirth rate. As 50% of women test positive, 22,272 women would need to be approached and tested [26]. Another alternative is to use a surrogate outcome such as a composite poor perinatal outcome (e.g. metabolic acidosis at birth, admission to NICE, small for gestational age infant), 1,447 participants in each arm would be required to demonstrate a 20% reduction in composite outcome. As there are approximately 14,000 women who consult with RFM after 36 weeks' gestation (and thus who would be eligible for the study), a study with stillbirth as the sole primary outcome would be unfeasible in the UK alone. However, using a composite primary outcome or randomisation after testing approach appropriate recruitment would be achievable. Novel trial designs such as stepped-wedge cluster randomised controlled trials (where an intervention is introduced to units in a random step-wise manner) offer more robust methodology than historical case-control studies and may address difficulties in obtaining statistical power to demonstrate a reduction in stillbirths. The priorities for studies to inform care identified by the ISA CHNRI exercise were: (i) implementation of smoking cessation programmes as part of routine antenatal care, (ii) use of perinatal audit and facility quality improvement to reduce stillbirth rates, and (iii) the optimum mode and timing of birth for infants with FGR to reduce stillbirth and neonatal and infant mortality and severe morbidity [3].

Implementing change

For perinatal audit and research to prevent stillbirths, the findings must result in changes to guidelines and/or protocols which directly affect care. However, this process is not straightforward which can be illustrated using RFMs as an example, because suboptimal management has been identified as a factor in stillbirths [17]. A questionnaire study in 2008 demonstrated wide variation in clinical practice with regard to the management of reduced fetal movements [27]. In 2010, the Royal College of Obstetricians and Gynaecologists (RCOG) published a national evidence-based guideline which incorporated the findings from two important studies. These were a randomised-controlled trial which demonstrated that kick-counting using an alarm limit of 10 movements in 12 hours did not reduce the number of stillbirths and a 'before and after' study describing a quality improvement project in Norway which reduced stillbirths from 3.0 per 1,000 to 2.0 per 1,000. A follow-up study in 2011–2012 found that the recommendations developed from this evidence were not incorporated into the majority of local guidelines, and 11% of units continued to recommend the use of kick counting [28]. This finding does not seem to be limited to local guidelines, as even national guidelines in maternity care show significant variation in their recommendations and quality [29]. This key element of stillbirth prevention is often overlooked, but the science of implementing change is a growing field of research, and the best methods to improve clinical practice and reduce stillbirth need to be identified.

PREVENTING STILLBIRTHS – A VISION FOR 2020

In the stillbirth series published in the Lancet in 2011 the authors called upon countries with a stillbirth rate less than 5.0 per 1,000 births (after 28 weeks) to eradicate preventable stillbirths and reduce stillbirths resulting from health inequalities by 2020. The lack of reduction in the stillbirth rate in the UK over the last two decades, coupled with evidence that the UK has one of the highest stillbirth rates in high-income countries provides impetus to address this issue. Prevention of stillbirth requires a raft of measures to improve the health and wellbeing of women before and during pregnancy. Due to its multifactorial nature there is no 'magic bullet' that will prevent stillbirth. Instead efforts should be directed to introducing measures that are known to be effective and improving understanding of the causes of stillbirth. Interventions and strategies identified as priority areas for stillbirth prevention are shown in **Table 6.1**.

Preconception care is recommended for all women, particularly those with pre-existing medical disorders such as diabetes, so that maternal health can be optimised prior to pregnancy. The provision of antenatal care to social disadvantaged and minority groups needs to be addressed. Maternity care should be accessible to all, overcoming organisation, personal and financial barriers to engaging in antenatal care. To this end the NICE have produced a guideline for the care of women with complex social factors providing models of pregnancy care for women who may be excluded from high-quality antenatal care [30].

Antenatal care needs to detect women at increased risk of stillbirth and optimise their management. All women should have a dating scan at 10–12 weeks' gestation to provide a baseline for assessing fetal growth and to prevent prolonged pregnancy beyond 42 completed weeks. Women with pre-existing medical complications such as diabetes and hypertension should be managed in specialist antenatal clinics with multidisciplinary input from clinicians and obstetricians. The control of these conditions is closely related

Table 6.1 Interventions and strategies to address priority areas for stillbirth prevention*

Area of focus	Strategies
Improvement of general health of women before, during and after pregnancy	Culturally appropriate preconception care for women throughout reproductive years to ensure adequate folic acid intake, optimum weight and diet, health education regarding smoking cessation, alcohol intake and substance misuse
Detection and management of women at increased risk of stillbirth	All women should have accurate dating of pregnancy
Socially excluded women	Culturally appropriate accessible antenatal care
Diabetes/overweight/obesity	Screening for complications and individualised care plan including dietician and postpartum weight management, exercise plan, routine weighing at first visit
Smoking, alcohol and illicit drug use	Screening for smoking, alcohol and substance misuse. Referral to appropriate services including smoking cessation
Screening for placental insufficiency/FGR	Screening for risk factors, ultrasound measurement of fetal growth for women at increased risk of FGR; increased awareness of RFM and timely evaluation. Use of umbilical artery Doppler in high-risk pregnancies. Low dose aspirin in those at increased risk of pre-eclampsia/FGR
Prolonged pregnancy	Induction of labour after 41 weeks' gestation
Improvement of information and standards of maternity care	Implementation of national perinatal mortality audit programmes (or MBRRACE) Improve data access with systems to more effectively use routinely collected data, consensus on a minimum dataset to monitor pregnancy outcomes Implement international classification systems to enable comparisons between units, regions and countries High-quality stillbirth investigation protocol, including placental histopathology for all stillbirths. Access to high-quality postmortem, chromosomal analysis and Kleihauer for all parents after stillbirth if they wish

FGR, fetal growth restriction; RFM, reduced fetal movements.
*Adapted from Flenady et al. Lancet 2011; 377:1703–1717.

to pregnancy outcome and should be optimised. Of all the potentially modifiable risk factors associated with stillbirth, cigarette smoking is most amenable to intervention during pregnancy. Guidelines from the NICE recommend a comprehensive approach to detection and treatment for women who smoke during pregnancy [31].

As FGR is the most commonly associated factor with stillbirth in high-income countries, improvement in screening for FGR coupled with appropriate timing of delivery is likely to reduce stillbirth. Clinicians should appreciate the importance of screening for FGR while acknowledging the limitations of current methods to do so; abdominal palpation misses a significant proportion of FGR fetuses, even when combined with a customised growth chart [32]. Therefore, the risk factors for FGR should be reviewed at the beginning of pregnancy and those at increased risk should have serial scans to assess fetal growth and screen for placental insufficiency [32]. In women with high-risk pregnancies, umbilical artery Doppler reduces perinatal mortality [33].

It is important that risk-status is re-evaluated at each contact with maternity services. Reduced fetal movements, a common reason for presentation in late pregnancy, is associated with an increased risk of FGR and stillbirth [25]. There is some evidence that increased education of women and care providers coupled with appropriate investigation and intervention might reduce the risk of stillbirth. This is currently being evaluated in a clinical trial being conducted in the UK [37].

The timing of delivery should also be optimised to reduce perinatal mortality. A systematic review on induction of labour at or beyond 41 weeks' gestation reduced perinatal mortality compared to expectant management [34]. Data suggests that offering induction of labour at 39 40 weeks in women with advanced maternal age ≥40 years would reduce the stillbirth rate for this group [35].

To ensure on-going improvements in stillbirth rates, the quality of information available to determine the cause of stillbirths and methods to assess the quality of care provided both need to be improved. In the UK, MBRRACE are now responsible for national data collection, but individual units must also review stillbirths locally, to understand causes of stillbirth in their units and identify potential deficiencies in care. Approaching parents after the death of their child to discuss investigations to determine a potential cause is not easy. Indeed, a significant proportion of obstetricians and midwives receive insufficient training in this area resulting in incomplete knowledge which may affect the accuracy of counselling bereaved parents [36]. Identifying the cause of stillbirth is important to parents [6,36], and all should have access to postmortem, placental histological examination, chromosomal analysis and Kleihauer testing as a minimum should they wish. In response to data from perinatal audit and case reviews maternity units should develop action plans to reduce stillbirths, the impact of which are reassessed in future audits.

CONCLUSION

A significant proportion of stillbirths in the UK are preventable, with better understanding of the causes of stillbirth leading to development and implementation of evidence-based interventions the stillbirth rate could be decreased further to be in line with other European countries such as the Netherlands and Norway. This needs to be augmented by research efforts to understand why stillbirths occur in the absence of apparent risk-factors and to develop better methods to identify FGR and placental insufficiency facilitating appropriate interventions.

Key points for clinical practice

- Stillbirth affects 1:200 pregnancies in the UK, one of the highest rates in high-income countries. Stillbirth has an important and enduring health, economic and social impact.
- Prevention of stillbirth requires a good understanding of relevant causes of stillbirth which are amenable to intervention.
- Perinatal audit needs to be completed locally and nationally and audit cycles completed to evaluate improvements in care.
- Perinatal audit requires high-quality data with as much relevant information as possible obtained from investigations most likely to find a cause of stillbirth.
- Investigations should be offered to determine a cause of stillbirth; these should be targeted to those most likely to find useful information for parents and clinicians.
- Epidemiological studies have highlighted risk factors for stillbirth, although few are sufficiently strong to significantly reduce the numbers of stillbirth in isolation.
- Stillbirth is under-researched compared to other pregnancy complications, more robust studies are required to understand and prevent stillbirth.
- Undertaking studies where the prevention of stillbirth is the primary goal is important, but requires large numbers or advanced clinical trials methods.
- On-going research projects aim to look at smoking cessation, advanced maternal age and the management of reduced fetal movements.
- Research and guidance needs to be translated into changes in clinical practice.

REFERENCES

1. Cousens S, Blencowe H, Stanton C, et al. National, regional, and worldwide estimates of stillbirth rates in 2009 with trends since 1995: a systematic analysis. Lancet 2011; 377:1319–1330.
2. Lawn JE, Blencowe H, Pattinson R, et al. Stillbirths: Where? When? Why? How to make the data count? Lancet 2011; 377:1448–1463.
3. Flenady V, Middleton P, Smith GC, et al. Stillbirths: the way forward in high-income countries. Lancet 2011; 377:1703–1717.
4. Confidential Enquiry into Maternal and Child Health. Perinatal mortality 2008: England, Wales and Northern Ireland. London: Centre for Enquiries into Maternal and Child Health, 2010.
5. Stock SJ, Ferguson E, Duffy A, et al. Outcomes of elective induction of labour compared with expectant management: population based study. BMJ 2012; 344:e2838.
6. Downe S, Schmidt E, Kingdon C, et al. Bereaved parents' experience of stillbirth in UK hospitals: a qualitative interview study. BMJ Open 2013; 3(2).
7. Reddy UM. Prediction and prevention of recurrent stillbirth. Obstet Gynecol 2007; 110:1151–1164.
8. Samueloff A, Xenakis EM, Berkus MD, et al. Recurrent stillbirth. Significance and characteristics. J Reprod Med 1993; 38:883–886.
9A. Michalski ST, Porter J, Pauli RM. Costs and consequences of comprehensive stillbirth assessment. Am J Obstet Gynecol 2002; 186:1027–1034.
9B. Mistry H, Heazell AE, Vincent O, et al. A structured review and exploration of the healthcare costs associated with stillbirth and a subsequent pregnancy in England and Wales. BMC Pregnancy Childbirth 2013; 13:236.
10. National Institute for Health and Clinical Excellence (NICE). Clinical guideline 63 – diabetes in pregnancy: management of diabetes and its complications from pre-conception to the postnatal period. London: NICE, 2008.
11. Mead J. Stillbirth claims. Clinical Risk 2010; 16:77–80.
12. Goldenberg RL, McClure EM, Bhutta ZA, et al. Stillbirths: the vision for 2020. Lancet 2011; 377:1798–1805.

13. Dunn PM, McIlwaine G. Perinatal AUDIT: A report produced for the European Association of Perinatal Medicine. New York: Parthenon 1996.
14. Dahl LB, Berge LN, Dramsdahl H, et al. Antenatal, neonatal and post neonatal deaths evaluated by medical audit. A population-based study in northern Norway – 1976 to 1997. Acta Obstet Gynecol Scand 2000; 79:1075–1082.
15. Butler NR, Bonham DG. Perinatal mortality: the first report of the 1958 British Perinatal mortality survey. London: E and S Livingstone, 1963.
16. Alderliesten ME, Stronks K, Bonsel GJ, et al. Design and evaluation of a regional perinatal audit. Eur J Obstet Gynecol Reprod Biol 2008; 137:141–145.
17. Confidential enquiry into stillbirths and deaths in infancy. 8th Annual Report. London: Maternal and Child Health Research Consortium, 2001.
18. Shaw B, Cheater F, Baker R, et al. Tailored interventions to overcome identified barriers to change: effects on professional practice and health care outcomes. Cochrane Database Syst Rev 2005:CD005470.
19. Cockerill R, Whitworth MK, Heazell AE. Do medical certificates of stillbirth provide accurate and useful information regarding the cause of death? Paediatr Perinat Epidemiol 2012; 26:117–123.
20. Korteweg FJ, Erwich JJ, Timmer A, et al. Evaluation of 1025 fetal deaths: proposed diagnostic workup. Am J Obstet Gynecol 2012; 206:53 e1-12.
21. Royal College of Obstetricians and Gynaecologists (RCOG). Green-Top Guideline 55 – Late Intrauterine Fetal Death and Stillbirth. London: RCOG, 2010.
22. Vergani P, Cozzolino S, Pozzi E, et al. Identifying the causes of stillbirth: a comparison of four classification systems. Am J Obstet Gynaecol 2008; 199:319 e1–4.
23. Stacey T, Thompson JM, Mitchell EA, et al. Association between maternal sleep practices and risk of late stillbirth: a case-control study. BMJ 2011; 342:d3403.
24. Haws RA, Yakoob MY, Soomro T, et al. Reducing stillbirths: screening and monitoring during pregnancy and labour. BMC Pregnancy Childbirth 2009; 9:S5.
25. Heazell AE, Frøen JF. Methods of fetal movement counting and the detection of fetal compromise. J Obstet Gynaecol 2008; 28:147–154.
26. Smith GCS. Scientific Advisory committee opinion paper 20 – evaluating new screening methodologies. London: Royal College of Obstetricians and Gynaecologists, 2010.
27. Heazell AE, Green M, Wright C, et al. Midwives' and obstetricians' knowledge and management of women presenting with decreased fetal movements. Acta Obstet Gynecol Scand 2008: 331–339.
28. Jones F, Saunders A, Heazell AE, et al. Reduced fetal movements – has RCOG guidance been translated into practice? Arch Dis Child Fetal Neonatal ED 2013; 98:A101.
29. Winther LP, Mitchell AU, Moller AM. Inconsistencies in clinical guidelines for obstetric anaesthesia for caesarean section: a comparison of the Danish, English, American, and German guidelines with regard to developmental quality and guideline content. Acta Anaesthesiol Scand 2013; 57:141–149.
30. National Institute for Health and Clinical Excellence (NICE). Clinical Guideline 110: Pregnancy and Complex Social Factors London: NICE, 2010.
31. National Institute for Health and Clinical Excellence (NICE). Clinical Guideline 26 – Quitting smoking in pregnancy and following childbirth. London: National Institute for Health and Clinical Excellence, 2010.
32. Royal College Of Obstetricians and Gynaecologists. The investigation and management of the small-for-gestational-age fetus. London: RCOG, 2013.
33. Alfirevic Z, Stampalija T, Gyte GM. Fetal and umbilical Doppler ultrasound in high-risk pregnancies. Cochrane Database Syst Rev 2010:CD007529.
34. Gulmezoglu AM, Crowther CA, Middleton P. Induction of labour for improving birth outcomes for women at or beyond term. Cochrane Database Syst Rev 2006:CD004945.
35. Royal College of Obstetricians and Gynaecologists (RCOG). Scientific Impact Paper 34 – Induction of Labour at Term in Older Mothers. London: RCOG, 2013.
36. Heazell A, McLaughlin MJ, Schmidt E, et al. A difficult conversation? The views and experiences of parents and professionals on the consent process for perinatal postmortem after stillbirth. BJOG 2012; 119:987–997.
37. Promoting awareness fetal movements to reduce fetal mortality stillbirth, a stepped wedge cluster randomised trial (AFFIRM). Clinical Trials Ref NCT01777022. http://www.clinicaltrials.gov/ct2/show/NCT01777022.

Chapter 7

Management of maternal cardiac disease in pregnancy

Julia Zöllner, Philip J Steer

INTRODUCTION

Heart disease in pregnancy is the leading cause of indirect maternal mortality in the United Kingdom (UK). In the last confidential enquiries into maternal deaths report in the UK [1], 53 women died from heart disease, demonstrating a rising trend in mortalities over the past 20 years [1]. Due to the dramatic advances in open heart surgery in the 1960s and 1970s, women with congenital heart disease (CHD) are now able to survive to childbearing age and choose to get pregnant. Despite an increased risk of obstetric and neonatal complications, they can achieve good pregnancy outcomes provided that they are managed in a multidisciplinary team setting and offered careful monitoring. The increase in maternal death rates in the UK from 7.3 per 100,000 in the triennium ending in 1984 to 23.1 per 100,000 in the triennium ending in 2008 was not however due to congenital heart disease (rates actually fell from 2.6 to 1.3 per 100,000) but to a dramatic increase in acquired heart disease (death rates increased from 7.3 to 23.1 per 100,000), (Figure 7.1). This rising incidence is likely attributable to changes in modern lifestyle including: the delay of pregnancy until later life, smoking, alcohol consumption, obesity and other chronic conditions. There has also been an increase in the incidence of rheumatic heart disease due to the increased proportion of pregnancies in women born overseas – 25.1% of all pregnancies in 2010, up from 12.1% in 1993. This phenomenon is being seen in many developed countries. It raises important questions as to how women, especially those with no previous health evaluations, presenting at their first antenatal check, should be assessed for occult cardiac disease [2].

In this chapter, we will discuss advances in the management of cardiac disease in pregnancy, both congenital and acquired. We will review clinical features, diagnosis and recent advances to care for women with heart disease in pregnancy.

Julia Zöllner MBBS BSc(Hons), Imperial College London, South Kensington Campus, London, UK. Email: j.zollner@imperial.ac.uk (for correspondence)

Philip J Steer BSc MBBS MD FRCOG FCOGSA(Hon), Imperial College London, UK. Email: p.steer@imperial.ac.uk

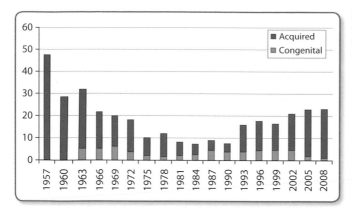

Figure 7.1 Maternal death rates from congenital and acquired heart disease over the last 50 years in the UK (rates per 100,000).

CARDIOVASCULAR CHANGES IN PREGNANCY

At the outset, it is important to have a basic understanding of the substantial cardiovascular alterations which occur to meet the increased maternal and fetal metabolic demands of a normal pregnancy. These changes occur early on in pregnancy and peak by the end of the second trimester. Circulating hormones such as oestrogens and prostaglandins and a low-resistance placental bed trigger a fall in the systemic and pulmonary vascular tone thereby creating a state of intravascular volume depletion. In compensation, plasma volume increases, leading to an increased stroke volume. To cope with this physiological stress, the maternal heart increases its compliance, contractility and size, thus modifying the function of the left ventricle – a condition commonly referred to as physiological cardiac hypertrophy. The heart valves increase in size, causing a higher incidence of valvular regurgitation. Overall, the maternal adaptation to pregnancy results in a 70% reduction in total vascular resistance (TVR), a 50% increase in cardiac output (CO) and a 40% increase in blood volume causing a dilutional 'anaemia'. Many cardiac lesions compromise, to a varying degree, the ability of the maternal heart to meet the demand for an increase in cardiac output. In some conditions a right-to-left shunt becomes more pronounced and results in worsening cyanosis [3, 4].

Women with known heart problems should receive pre-pregnancy counselling, be offered adequate contraception advice, and be encouraged to lead a healthy lifestyle. Such counselling should be given by an experienced cardiologist or obstetrician (preferably both, in a combined clinic) who has experience of dealing with heart disease in pregnancy. It is important that a detailed assessment of the woman's cardiac status is made, and the risks associated with pregnancy explained, prior to conception. The aim is to optimise, if necessary, the woman's cardiac condition prior to conceiving, to manage the expectations of her and her partner/family by explaining potential maternal and fetal risks, and plan the level of surveillance. For some women a pregnancy might be so high risk that it is inadvisable [3] but ultimately, modern practice is to respect and support a woman's informed decision.

CONGENITAL HEART DISEASE

The incidence of maternal CHD in pregnancy is increasing in the UK. This is partly explained by advances in surgical and medical therapies over the past few decades [5].

In the UK, each year about 1600 patients with complex CHD enter adulthood, of whom half are female. Many will plan to have their own families. They need to be counselled and screened for CHD in their own offspring; for the multigenetic syndromes such as Fallot's tetralogy the recurrence risk is generally between 3 and 5% (the overall population incidence of congenital cardiac disease at birth being 0.8%), while for single gene defects such as Marfan's syndrome, the recurrence risk is 50%. All women with known CHD are currently offered detailed antenatal fetal ultrasound screening by a paediatric cardiologist or similar specialist. However, most babies with CHD are born to mothers without cardiac disease themselves. A recent study reported a raised incidence of CHD in babies born to mothers with genetic and environmental risk factors such as maternal obesity and diabetes, advanced maternal and paternal age at conception, maternal smoking during pregnancy, maternal urinary tract infections and exposure to non-fertility medication [6]. This raises the question of whether more detailed second trimester screening to identify CHD should be offered to those pregnant patients who have these risk factors because early detection improves neonatal outcomes [7].

Congenital heart disease patients comprise the majority of the workload in a cardiac antenatal clinic, and warrant careful surveillance, as they are at increased risk of maternal, fetal and neonatal complications. The commonest serious cardiac complications are pulmonary oedema, arrhythmia, and stroke, and these are also the main causes of mortality [8]. Fetal complications include preterm birth, fetal growth restriction and stillbirth [9]. Poor antenatal cardiovascular status is an important predictor of adverse outcomes. Risk factors associated with poor outcomes in pregnancy include:
- Poor functional class (New York Heart Association classification > II)
- Cyanosis (Sao_2 < 90%)
- Systemic ventricular ejection fraction <40%
- Prior cardiovascular event (arrhythmia, pulmonary oedema, stroke or transient ischaemic attack)

The spectrum of CHD lesions and their possible surgical repairs is vast. Furthermore, the severity of functional impairment shows considerable variation within the same condition, explaining the need for individualised pre-pregnancy counselling [9]. Apart from the anatomical lesion itself, one must also consider other complicating disorders, such as pulmonary disease and in particular pulmonary hypertension. Thorne et al. [10] devised four groups according to their level of risk; mild, moderate, severe and extreme risk groups (Table 7.1). These groups have subsequently been further adapted by the European Society of Cardiology (ESC) into comprehensive disease descriptions and have been incorporated in their latest guidelines (Table 7.2) [11]. However, a simple anatomical description of the lesion is insufficient to categorise risk because functional status and previous related adverse events, as listed above, also need to be taken into account. The expected adverse cardiac event rate during pregnancy increases with the number of additional risk factors; 0, 1 or >1 of these increase the risk by 5%, 27% and 75% respectively [8].

Throughout the antenatal period careful attention needs to be paid to any signs of de-compensating heart function. Sign and symptoms of clinical deterioration during pregnancy include:
- Decreased exercise tolerance
- Increased palpitations
- Irregular pulse
- Change in previous heart murmur
- Increased blood pressure

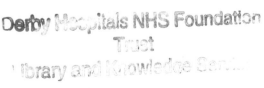

Table 7.1 Classification of maternal cardiovascular risk

Class	Risk	Notes
I	No noticeable increased risk in regards to maternal mortally and no/mild increased risk in morbidity	
II	A small increased risk in mortality or a moderate increase in morbidity	
III	A significant increased risk of maternal mortality or severe morbidity	Careful pre-pregnancy counselling required. If pregnancy is decided upon, careful specialist monitoring is required
IV	An extremely high risk of maternal mortality or severe morbidity; pregnancy contraindicated	As for notes on class III, but pregnancy should strongly be advised against

Modified from WHO classification of maternal cardiovascular risk [11]
WHO, World Health Organization.

Table 7.2 Application of classification of maternal cardiovascular risk

WHO risk class	Example of heart conditions
WHO I	Uncomplicated, small or mild: • Pulmonary stenosis • Ventricular septal defect • Patent ductus arteriosus • Mitral valve prolapse with no more than trivial mitral regurgitation Successfully repaired simple lesion: • Ostium secundum atrial septal defect • Ventricular septal defect • Patent ductus arteriosus • Total anomalous pulmonary venous drainage Isolated ventricular extrasystoles and atrial ectopic beats
WHO II (If otherwise well and uncomplicated)	Un-operated atrial septal defects Repaired tetralogy of Fallot Most arrhythmias
WHO II–III (depending on individual)	Mild left ventricular impairment Hypertrophic cardiomyopathy Native or tissue valvular heart disease not considered WHO 4 Marfan syndrome without aortic dilatation Heart transplantation
WHO III	Mechanical valve Systemic right ventricle (e.g. congenitally corrected transposition, simple transposition post Mustard or Senning repair) Post Fontan operation Cyanotic heart disease Other complex congenital heart disease
WHO IV (pregnancy contraindicated)	Pulmonary arterial hypertension of any cause Severe systemic ventricular dysfunction: NYHA III-IV or LVEF <30% Previous peripartum cardiomyopathy with any residual impairment of left ventricular function Severe left heart obstruction Marfan syndrome with aorta dilated >40 mm

Modified from WHO application of classification of maternal cardiovascular risk [11]
LVEF, left ventricular ejection fraction; NYHA, New York Heart Association; WHO, World Health Organization.

- Decreased oxygen saturation
- Added sounds on auscultation of the lungs
- Increasing ankle oedema

It is important that patients are seen by the same clinician at every antenatal check-up so that any significant changes can be detected early, allowing for timely intervention. Regular fetal growth scans are recommended for any woman with cyanosis or significant impairment of cardiac output, or whose baby is clinically small. Initially, appointments should be scheduled for every 2–3 weeks. From 28 weeks' gestation, check-ups should be every week. Depending on the cardiac severity, and the distance of her home from the hospital, women may need to be admitted prior to delivery and to await labour, spontaneous or induced, as an in-patient. Regular multi-disciplinary meetings discussing the overall management of the patients are important, most commonly in the form of a joint cardiac clinic hosted by senior cardiologists and obstetricians.

ACQUIRED HEART DISEASE

Acute myocardial infarction

Although acute myocardial infarction (AMI) and ischaemic heart disease (IHD) in pregnancy is rare, it contributes to one-fifth of all cardiac related deaths in the UK [1]. A recent UK Obstetric Surveillance System (UKOSS) report [12] estimated the incidence of pregnancy-related AMI at 0.7 per 100,000 maternities. The reported incidence in other industrialised countries varies between 1.3 and 6.7 per 100,000 births. It is likely that the incidence of acquired heart disease is increasing [12]. In the last centre for maternal and child enquiries (CMACE), UK report [1], coronary atheroma was the underlying pathology in 50% of the women who died from myocardial infarction (MI) [1]. In non-fatal cases of AMI the aetiologies were coronary artery dissection and coronary arterial thrombosis, but AMI can occur even with normal coronary arteries. Over three-quarters of cases occurred in the latter half of pregnancy or postpartum [12]. In contrast to survivors, none of the women who died had known pre-existing heart disease, demonstrating the need for addressing risk factors preconception if possible, and if not, identifying them as early as possible in the antenatal clinic [9]. These conclusions are reinforced by a Dutch cohort study published in 2013 [13]. Pregnancy itself increases the risk of AMI by 3–4 times due to the haemodynamic changes and hypercoagulability induced by pregnancy [14, 15]. Increased maternal age also increases the risk. In vitro fertilisation (IVF) enables women to achieve pregnancies in their 40s (or even 50s and beyond), increasing their risk of AMI 30-fold compared to women below the age of 20 years [14]. Lifestyle factors such as obesity and smoking, as well as pre-existing conditions including hypertension, diabetes and hyperlipidaemia, further add to risk. Obstetric risk factors include pre-eclampsia, postpartum infection, postpartum haemorrhage and twin pregnancy [12, 14].

Symptoms and signs can be difficult to recognise in pregnancy as they can overlap with those normal in pregnancy (**Table 7.3**). A high level of suspicion is therefore necessary. Chest pain requires prompt investigation with an electrocardiogram (ECG) and measurement of cardiac enzymes (preferably cardiac troponins as their level is not affected by uterine contractions or other cell breakdown that occurs through pregnancy and labour) [16]. **Table 7.4** compares normal ECG changes in pregnancy with those occurring in an evolving AMI [17, 18]. In the UK, the management of AMI in pregnancy, both medical

Table 7.3 Signs and symptoms of normal versus heart disease in pregnancy

Associated with normal pregnancy

1. Fatigue
2. Exertional dyspnoea
3. Palpitation (re-entry tachycardia, atrial and ventricular premature beats)
4. Elevated jugular venous pressure
5. Sinus tachycardia 10–15% above normal heart rate
6. Full volume pulse
7. Third heart sound
8. Systolic flow murmur
9. Pedal oedema

Associated with cardiac pathology

1. Chest pain
2. Severe breathlessness, orthopnoea, paroxysmal nocturnal dyspnoea, cough
3. Atrial flutter or fibrillation, ventricular tachycardia
4. Systemic hypotension
5. Sinus tachycardia > 15% above normal heart rate
6. Fourth heart sound
7. Pulmonary oedema
8. Pleural effusion

Modified from Thorne S [4]

Table 7.4 Diagnosis of acute myocardial infarction (MI) and normal ECG changes in pregnancy

Criteria for acute, evolving or recent MI
Either one of the following criteria satisfy the diagnosis:

1. Typical rise and gradual fall (troponin) with at least one of the following:

    a. Ischaemic symptoms

    b. Development of pathologic Q waves on the ECG

    c. ECG changes indicative of ischaemia (ST segment elevation or depression), or

    d. Coronary artery intervention (e.g. coronary angioplasty)

2. Pathologic findings of an acute MI

Commonly found ECG changes in uncomplicated pregnancy:

1. Left or right axis deviation
2. Small Q waves in lead III
3. T wave inversion
4. Increased R/S ratio in leads V1 and V2

and surgical, is highly variable as clear guidelines are lacking [12]. Whichever treatment is chosen, it needs to be given promptly if it is to reduce the morbidity and mortality of both mother and fetus [18]. The choice of treatment is dependent on the stage of pregnancy or puerperium. The ESC recommends coronary angiography with the possibility of percutaneous coronary intervention (PCI) as first line management during the acute phase of ST elevation. PCI is the only effective treatment when the aetiology is coronary artery dissection. Bare metal stents are most commonly used, rather than drug eluting stents, as the safety of the latter in pregnancy is still unknown. Similarly, dual antiplatelet therapy such as aspirin and clopidogrel should be avoided as its safety is not yet established. Thrombolytic therapy is only recommended for life threatening situations where PCI is not available [11]. The complication rate of thrombolytic therapy is about 1% and most reports of its use in pregnancy have been in the treatment of pulmonary embolism [19]. In non-ST elevation MI, PCI can be considered but watchful waiting and commencement of medical treatment can be appropriate if the patient is in a stable condition [11]. Unfortunately, current practice in the UK is that less than two thirds of patients undergo angiography, with only half of these receiving coronary angioplasty and stenting. This suggests room for improvement. **Table 7.5** summarises the key points in the management of AMI in pregnancy [12].

The options for medical treatment are limited by pregnancy. Drug safety is not well-established for many new medications (e.g. glycoprotein IIb/IIIa inhibitors, bivalirudin, prasugrel and ticagrelor), and they are therefore not currently recommended in pregnancy. ACE inhibitors, angiotensin receptor blockers (ARBs), renin inhibitors and statins are currently contraindicated during pregnancy [11], as they are associated with teratogenicity [20–22]. The use of beta-blockers, aspirin, diuretics or hydralazine is more established and they are considered generally safe. Although beta-blockers probably cause some fetal growth restriction, their benefits may outweigh this risk. It is currently advised that clopidogrel is used cautiously and for the shortest period possible, due to concerns about possible harm to the fetus and the risk of bleeding, especially around the time of delivery [21].

PERIPARTUM CARDIOMYOPATHY

Peripartum cardiomyopathy (PPCM) is a rare but life-threatening condition resulting in significant long-term cardiac sequelae. It is defined by left ventricular systolic dysfunction, with an ejection fraction below 45%, in the absence of any underlying heart disease or other identifiable cause occurring mainly towards the end of pregnancy or within the early postpartum period. The incidence is estimated at 1 in 3000 to 4000 pregnancies. The 7-year case fatality rate in a recent population-based study was 16.5%, i.e. 1 in 6 women died. A four-fold increased prevalence has been reported in black women, and women over the age of 35 years [23]. Other known risk factors include: obesity, smoking, lower socioeconomic status, chronic hypertension, twin pregnancy, tocolytic therapy and pre-eclampsia.

Recent advances have shed some light on the possible molecular mechanisms underlying PPCM. There is evidence suggesting that oxidative stress and consequential endothelial dysfunction is a component of the pathophysiological process, which partly explains its strong association with pre-eclampsia. It appears that 16 kDa prolactin (16-kDa PRL), a

Table 7.5 Key points in the management of acute myocardial infarction in pregnancy
Principles of management are the same as in non-pregnant patients
History taking: relevant symptoms, elicit characteristic signs
Investigations: ECG, cardiac enzymes (troponin I)
Treatment: coronary angiography +/− PCI. Supportive medical therapy such as drug treatment Drug treatment should only be commenced in pregnant patients under specialist guidance

cleavage product of prolactin during oxidative stress, is an antiangiogenic, proapoptotic, and proinflammatory molecule [24]. Its effects are mediated by 16-kDa PRL inhibiting mitogen-activated protein kinase which results in inhibition of endothelial cell proliferation by impairing vessel maturation and inhibiting proliferation, migration, and vasodilatation. Recent novel findings demonstrated that treatment with bromocriptine (an inhibitor of prolactin secretion) in an animal model successfully prevented the onset of disease. Since then, human clinical experience has suggested that bromocriptine has beneficial effects, changing PPCMs bleak prognosis. Further experimental and clinical evidence to support this, such as from larger clinical trials, is needed.

Peripartum cardiomyopathy presents acutely and delay in diagnosis can be detrimental. Early recognition by clinicians is important but its early symptoms and signs can be confused with those of normal pregnancy: fatigue, mild shortness of breath and oedema. A careful clinical assessment including history and examination is crucial in all women with such symptoms. **Table 7.6** summarises the symptoms and signs, investigation findings and management of PPCM. Birth should be vaginal where possible, to avoid the additional stress of surgical delivery. The recurrence risk of PPCM is high, about 30–50%, particularly in women who do not recover their left ventricular function following

Table 7.6 Investigation, diagnosis and management of peripartum cardiomyopathy	
DIAGNOSIS, INVESTIGATION AND MANAGEMENT OF PPCM	
The symptoms are of acute heart failure presenting in previously healthy women: 1. Acute dyspnoea 2. Rapidly increasing exercise intolerance 3. Cough 4. Orthopnoea	The following symptoms may also occur: 1. Abdominal discomfort 2. Pleuritic chest pain 3. Palpitations
Investigations and typical findings	
ECG	Commonly normal, but sinus tachycardia and T-wave abnormalities may occur
Blood Samples	C-reactive protein is ↑, BNP ↑↑ (Markers of oxidative stress: oxidized LDL ↑, interferon gamma ↑)
Chest X-ray	Can show cardiomegaly, venous congestion & pleural effusion
Echocardiogram	LVEF < 45%, LV dilatation common, elevated LV filling pressure, atrioventricular valve regurgitation, LV thrombus
Cardiac Magnetic Resonance Imaging	A new useful tool, although only case reports describing its use in PPCM at present
Management	
First Line drug therapy of cardiomyopathy in non-pregnant patients comprises:	Beta-blockers (Metoprolol), ACE-Inhibitors or ARBs and diuretics
Alternative management in pregnancy	Hydralazine and nitrates can be used instead of ACE inhibitors, which are contraindicated in pregnancy.
Bromocriptine	Can be considered
Anticoagulation	Advisable if marked cardiomegaly and reduced EF
Adapted from Hilfiker-Kleiner et al. [24] PPCM; peripartum cardiomyopathy, LVEF; left ventricular ejection, ACE; angiotensin-converting enzyme	

pregnancy. Advice regarding further pregnancies therefore requires careful sequential assessment of cardiac function in the year or two following the affected pregnancy. Recent advances in PPCM and joint international registries hopefully will further our understanding and provide better guidance in the near future.

MARFAN SYNDROME IN PREGNANCY

Marfan syndrome (MFS) is an autosomal dominant inherited connective tissue disorder affecting 1 in 5000 of the population. Pregnancy is associated with an increased risk of aortic dissection because of its hormonal and haemodynamic changes. The risk of aortic dissection or other serious complications is about 1% in women with minimal cardiovascular risk factors and an aortic root dilation of <4 cm, but rises to as high as 10% as the aortic root diameter increases. Although dissection is rare, a completely safe diameter does not exist as dissection can occur even with an apparently normal root. The European Society of Cardiology recommends against pregnancy if the root diameter is over 4.5 cm [11].

A recent prospective study [25] looking at the immediate and long-term impact of pregnancy on aortic growth rate and mortality found that risk factors for adverse cardiovascular outcome included not only larger aortic size, but also a greater than average rate of aortic dilatation during pregnancy, more than one pregnancy, lack of beta-blockers protection during pregnancy, and poor antenatal care. Aortic root diameter did not always return to baseline following pregnancy. Further, elective aortic surgery during long-term follow up was higher in those who had had a pregnancy, compared to nulligravid women. However, no serious complications were encountered during pregnancy in women with an aortic root of <4.5 cm [25]. Our own experience of 16 patients [26] showed that most women with MFS appear to go through pregnancy uneventfully. However, two patients developed left ventricular dysfunction on echocardiographic evaluation. The reasons for this remain unclear. Both patients recovered promptly within 6 weeks of giving birth. We suggest that in subsequent pregnancies in these women, it will be important to monitor their ventricular function closely. The recommended management of MFS in pregnancy includes rigorous blood pressure monitoring and control, the use of beta-blockers in all women even when normotensive and regular echocardiographic monitoring. Delivery strategies should be aimed at minimising haemodynamic changes and ideally include epidural anaesthesia for labour and assisted vaginal delivery [25]. Although the use of beta-blockers in pregnancy is generally safe, there is now emerging evidence that they are associated with small for dates babies and so careful ultrasound monitoring of growth is necessary [27]. Women with MFS require care from a team of experienced obstetricians and cardiologists. Without preimplantation genetic diagnosis (over 80% will have an identifiable fibrillin gene mutation) and selective replacement of unaffected IVF embryos, the incidence of MFS in the fetus is 50% and therefore detailed counselling of the mother prior to the start of pregnancy is essential.

PULMONARY ARTERIAL HYPERTENSION

Pulmonary arterial hypertension (PAH), although a rare condition, poses a major risk in pregnancy. It is defined in non-pregnant women by the presence of a mean pulmonary artery pressure of >25 mmHg at rest or >30 mmHg on exercise in the absence of a left-to-right shunt. The incidence is estimated at 1.1 per 100,000 maternities. Common causes are primary (idiopathic) PAH, Eisenmenger's syndrome, or other underlying disease pathology such as cystic fibrosis and connective tissue disorders. Even as late as the end of the 20th century the prognosis was bleak, with maternal mortality rates as high as 40%. Although the risk remains high, advances in medical therapy since 2000 have likely improved the outcome (because the condition is rare, it is difficult to estimate even triennial mortality reliably) and the mortality rate in data published since 2003 varies from 16–30%. Most authors attribute the improved outcome to the introduction of improved therapies such as phosphodiesterase inhibitors, e.g. sildafenil and prostaglandin analogues and our own experience is consistent with this. In our case series of 12 pregnancies in nine women, there were no deaths during pregnancy but two deaths following delivery, one related to pre-eclampsia and one to arrhythmia (27). Remarkably in four patients the diagnosis was only made in their index pregnancy (around 24–36 weeks). In all of the 10 pregnancies since 2003, women have been anticoagulated with low-molecular weight heparin (prophylactic or therapeutic treatment depending on their thrombotic risk). Sildafenil was used in all nine pregnancies since 2007, and one required nebulised iloprost when her condition worsened. The majority were delivered by elective caesarean section between 32–39 weeks' gestation because of deterioration in maternal condition. We used general anaesthesia for logistical reasons but safe delivery using regional block has been reported by others [28, 29]. Most reported mortalities have occurred in the immediate post-natal period demonstrating the importance of following these patients closely after the delivery. In relation to long-term outcome, cardiac function does not appear to recover to baseline and therefore effective contraception should be strongly recommended to this group of patients. The development of multicentre registries [28, 30] to improve our understanding of this challenging condition must be a priority.

Key points for clinical practice

- Heart disease in pregnancy is the leading cause of indirect maternal mortality in the UK and of clinical importance.
- Heart disease in pregnancy is managed best in a multi-disciplinary team, led by an experienced obstetrician or cardiologist.
- Pre-pregnancy counselling in women with congenital heart disease, offering adequate contraception advice and optimising their cardiac status, is important.
- It is important to identify women at risk of acquired heart disease early in pregnancy and so symptoms such as chest pain and unusual shortness of breath should always be promptly and thoroughly investigated.
- The use of bromocriptine in the management of peripartum cardiomyopathy seems to have beneficial effects. The recurrence risk PPCM is high and careful evaluation of patient's left ventricular function following pregnancy is important.
- In Marfan's syndrome a completely safe root diameter does not exist but our own experience suggests that a diameter below 4.5 cm carries a risk which is acceptable to most women. In the absence of preimplantation genetic diagnosis, the recurrence rate in their offspring is 50% and therefore careful counselling prior to pregnancy is essential.
- Pulmonary hypertension in pregnancy is still associated with a high-morbidity and mortality rate. Recent advances such as the use of Sildafenil have improved the prognosis but care for these patients needs to be provided in specialist units.

REFERENCES

1. Centre for Maternal and Child Enquiries (CMACE). Saving Mothers' Lives: reviewing maternal deaths to make motherhood safer: 2006–2008 The eighth report of the confidential enquiries into maternal deaths in the United Kingdom. BJOG 2011; 118(suppl. 1):1-203.
2. Zöllner J, Curry R, Johnson M. The contribution of heart disease to maternal mortality. Curr Opin Obstet Gynecol 2012; 25:91–97.
3. Uebing A, Steer PJ, Yentis SM, et al. Pregnancy and congenital heart disease. BMJ 2006; 332:401–406.
4. Thorne S. Pregnancy in heart disease. Heart 2005; 90:450–456.
5. Uebing, A, Arvanitis P, Li W, et al. Effect of pregnancy on clinical status and ventricular function in women with heart disease. Int J Cardiol 2010; 139:50–59.
6. Fung A, Manlhiot C, Naik S, et al. Impact of prenatal risk factors on congenital heart disease in the current era. J Am Heart Assoc 2013; 2:e000064 .
7. Lapierre C, Rypens F, Grignon A, et al. Prenatal ultrasound screening of congenital heart disease in the general population: general concepts, guidelines, differential diagnoses. Ultrasound Q 2013; 29:111–124.
8. Siu S, Sermer M, Colman JM, et al. Prospective multicenter study of pregnancy outcomes in women with heart disease. Circulation 2001;104: 515–521.
9. Bowater S, Thorne S. Management of pregnancy in women with acquired and congenital heart disease. Postgrad Med J 2010; 86:100–105.
10. Thorne S, MacGregor A, Nelson-Piercy C. Risks of contracpetion and pregnancy in heart disease. Heart 2006; 92:1520–1525.
11. Regitz-Zagrosek V, Blomstrom Lundqvist C, Borghi C, et al. ESC Guidelines on the management of cardiovascular diseases in pregnancy: the Task Force on the Management of Cardiovascular Diseases during Pregnancy of the European Society of Cardiology (ESC). Eur Heart J 2011; 32:3147–3197.
12. Bush N, Nelson-Piercy C, Spark P, et al. Myocardial infarction in pregnancy and postpartum in the UK. Eur J Prev Cardiol 2013; 20:12–20.
13. Huisman CM, Roos-Hesselink JW, Duvekot JJ, et al. Incidence and predictors of maternal cardiovascular mortality and severe morbidity in the Netherlands: a prospective cohort study. PLoS One 2013; 8:e56494.
14. James A, Jamison M, Biswas M, et al. Acute myocardial infarction in pregnancy: a United States population-based study. Circulation 2006; 113:1564–1571.
15. Roth A, Elkayam U. Acute myocardial infarction associated with pregnancy. J Am Coll Cardiol 2008; 52:171–180.
16. Shade GJr, Ross G, Bever FN, et al. Troponin I in the diagnosis of acute myocardial infarction in pregnancy, labor, and post-partum. Am J Obstet Gynecol 2002; 187:1719–1720.
17. Myocardial infarction redefined. A consensus document of The Joint European Society of Cardiology/American College of Cardiology Committee for the Redefinition of Myocardial Infarction. Eur Heart J 2000; 21:1502–1513.
18. Kealey A. Coronary artery disease and myocardial infarction in pregnancy: a review of epidemiology, diagnosis, and medical and surgical management. Can J Cardiol. 2010; 26: e18–189.
19. Ahearn G, Hadjiliadis D, Govert J, et al. Massive pulmonary embolism during pregnancy successfully treated with recombinant tissue plasminogen activator: a case report and review of treatment options. Arch Intern Med 2002; 16:1221–1227.
20. Cooper W,Hernandez-Diaz S, Arbogast P, et al. Major Congenital malformations after first-trimester exposure to ACE inhibitors. N Engl J Med 2006;354:2443–2451.
21. Walfisch A, Al-maawali A, Moretti ME, et al. Teratogenicity of angiotensin converting enzyme inhibitors or receptor blockers. J Obstet Gynaecol 2011; 31:465–472.
22. Kusters DM, Lahsinoui HH, van de Post JA, et al. Statin use during pregnancy: a systematic review and meta-analysis. Expert Rev Cardiovasc Ther 2012; 10:363–378.
23. Harper MA, Meyer RE, Berg CJ. Peripartum cardiomyopathy: population-based birth prevalence and 7-year mortality. Obstet Gynecol 2012;120:1013–1019
24. Hilfiker-Kleiner D, Struman I, Hoch M, et al. 16-kDa prolactin and bromocriptine in postpartum cardiomyopathy. Curr Heart Fail Rep 2012; 9:174–182.
25. Donnelly RT, Pinto NM, Kocolas I, et al. The immediate and long-term impact of pregnancy on aortic growth rate and mortality in women with Marfan syndrome. J Am Coll Cardiol 2012; 60:224–229.
26. Curry R, Gelson E, Swan L, et al. Marfan syndrome and pregnancy – maternal and neonatal outcomes. BJOG 2014; Jan 13 doi: 10.1111/1471-0528.12515. [Epub ahead of print].
27. Meidahl Petersen K, Jimenez-Solem E, Andersen JT, et al. Beta-blocker treatment during pregnancy and adverse pregnancy outcomes: a nationwide population-based cohort study. BMJ Open 2012;2: pii: e001185.

28. Jaïs X, Olsson KM, Barbera JA, et al. Pregnancy outcomes in pulmonary arterial hypertension in the modern management era. Eur Respir J 2012; 40:881–885.
29. Duarte AG, Thomas S, Safdar Z, et al. Management of pulmonary arterial hypertension during pregnancy: a retrospective, multicenter experience. Chest 2013; 143:1330–1336.
30. Roos-Hesselink J, Ruys TP, Stein JI, et al. Outcome of pregnancy in patients with structural or ischaemic heart disease: results of a registry of the European Society of Cardiology. Eur Heart J 2013; 34:357–665.

Chapter 8

The role of breast cancer genes in gynaecological cancer

Angela George, Susana Banerjee

INTRODUCTION

There are multiple genes in which germline mutations have been associated with an increased susceptibility to breast cancer. These genes vary from rare, highly penetrant genes that confer a substantial risk of breast cancer to common gene mutations that confer only a small increased risk. This chapter will focus on the rare genes that confer a substantial increased risk of breast cancer, and the importance that such genes have for gynaecologists and oncologists specialising in gynaecological cancers.

INHERITED SUSCEPTIBILITY – BREAST/OVARIAN CANCER SYNDROMES

Familial (or hereditary) breast/ovarian cancer syndrome is caused by inherited germline mutations in several genes. Mutation carriers have increased risks of breast and/or ovarian cancer, although the proportion of cases may vary from family-to-family, with ovarian cancer predominating in some, and breast cancer in others. To date, the best known and most common genes implicated are breast cancer susceptibility genes 1 and 2 (*BRCA1* and *BRCA2*). Together, these account for ~5% of all breast cancer, and 10–15% of ovarian cancer.

BRCA1 was first identified in 1990 on the long arm of chromosome 17 (Ch17q21), following linkage studies of 23 Caucasian extended families, with multiple cases of early onset (<40 years) breast cancer [1]. Subsequent studies of five large families with multiple cases of breast and ovarian cancer showed linkage to the same site, providing the first genetic evidence of a link between ovarian and breast cancer [2]. *BRCA1* mutations were subsequently identified in families with ovarian cancer only (**Figure 8.1**).

BRCA2 was first localised in 1994, using 15 high-risk breast cancer families that had not been linked to *BRCA1*. Analysis of the families identified a common interval on the long arm of chromosome 13 (13q12-13) [13]. *BRCA2* associated families differed from *BRCA1*

Angela George MBChB FRACP, Gynaecology Unit, The Royal Marsden NHS Foundation Trust, UK. Email: angela.george@rmh.nhs.uk

Susana Banerjee MA MRCP PhD, Gynaecology Unit, The Royal Marsden NHS Foundation Trust, Surrey, UK. Email: susana.banerjee@rmh.nhs.uk (for correspondence)

associated families in that the strongest linkage included cases of male breast cancer, in addition to early-onset female breast cancer and ovarian cancer. *BRCA2* carriers also have an increased risk of pancreatic and prostate cancers (**Figure 8.2**).

The increased risk of developing cancer varies by gene. *BRCA1* mutations are associated with breast cancer risks of 39–87%, and an ovarian cancer risk of 39–66%. Those who carry a *BRCA2* mutation have similar breast cancer risks to *BRCA1* carriers, but an 11–27% risk of ovarian cancer. The average age of cancer diagnoses can also vary, with *BRCA1* carriers tending to be diagnosed at an earlier age that either *BRCA2* carriers, or non-carriers. The risk of developing a breast or ovarian cancer can also vary with the position of the mutation on the gene. Mutations that occur within a region on Exon 11 of *BRCA2*, known as the ovarian cancer cluster region (OCCR) have an ovarian:breast cancer ratio of 3:1 [4]. There is no similar clustering of mutations identified with *BRCA1*, but mutations in the 3' end of the gene are predominantly associated with breast cancer, while mutations towards the 5' end are associated with similar number of breast and ovarian cancers.

The frequency of *BRCA* mutations is dependent on the population mix. Whilst *BRCA* mutations are rare in general outbred populations, with rates of ~1/1000, higher rates have been identified is some countries, including Poland, Iceland and Russia. The highest rates have been identified in Ashkenazi Jews, where up to 2% of the population carry 1 of 3 recurrent (founder) mutations. These three mutations account for more than 97% of *BRCA* mutations found in Ashkenazi Jews, with two mutations in *BRCA1* (c.68_69delAG,

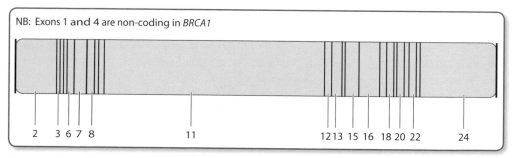

Figure 8.1 The *BRCA1* gene

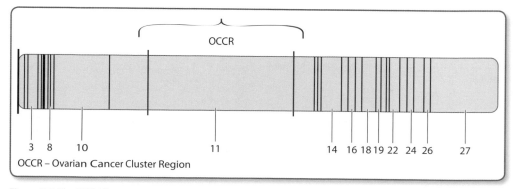

Figure 8.2 The *BRCA2* gene

c.5266dupC), and 1 in *BRCA2* (c.5946delT, situated within the OCCR) [5]. The higher population frequency rates also influence *BRCA* mutation frequency rates in ovarian or breast cancer studies, as those performed in areas with a high proportion of Ashkenazi Jewish participants have mutation frequency rates of up to 43%.

There are strong genotype and phenotype associations for *BRCA*-related breast cancers. Patients who carry a *BRCA1* mutation predominantly develop breast cancers which are negative for oestrogen receptors (ER), progesterone receptors (PR) and *HER2*. These tumours are referred to as triple negative tumours, and only account for 10% of breast cancer in non-carriers. In contrast, *BRCA2* carriers develop breast tumours with a similar receptor profile to non-carriers, with approximately 70% ER positive, 20% *HER2* positive, and 10% triple negative tumours.

BRCA TESTING IN CANCER PATIENTS

The choice of which women should undergo *BRCA* gene testing has historically been limited to women with a pre-specified higher likelihood of carrying a mutation and this is largely due to the cost and intensive nature of the *BRCA* testing process. The individual's risk can be estimated using programmes such as BRCAPRO and BOADICEA; scores such as the Manchester scoring system; or set clinical criteria, including features such as histological subtype, and age of diagnosis [6]. These methods utilise slightly different factors but most require a family history of cancer for patients to be considered at a high enough risk to warrant testing. It is now recognised that this approach may be missing ovarian cancer patients who carry a *BRCA* mutation, as large series of patients unselected for family history have demonstrated that up to half of ovarian cancer patients with a germline *BRCA* mutation do not have a significant family history [7]. These studies suggest that more widespread testing of women with breast and ovarian cancer is warranted, given the implications of finding a mutation for both the patient, and also their family members.

CLINICAL IMPLICATIONS OF *BRCA* MUTATIONS

Breast cancer

The knowledge of a patient's *BRCA* mutation status has several implications for the management of breast cancer. The majority of women diagnosed with breast cancer are offered mastectomy (+/– breast reconstruction), or breast-conserving surgery with a lumpectomy and breast irradiation. However, *BRCA* mutation carriers have an increased risk of second primary breast cancers, either in the contralateral breast, or in remaining ipsilateral breast tissue and may therefore choose to undergo more extensive surgery such as bilateral mastectomy to reduce this risk. In addition, women with *BRCA*-associated breast cancer have an increased risk of developing ovarian cancer and therefore prophylactic bilateral salpingo-oophorectomy needs to be discussed (see later). The *BRCA* mutation status may also influence the choice of systemic therapy for women with breast cancer. Platinum-based chemotherapy has been shown to have increased efficacy in *BRCA*-mutant breast cancer and clinical trials in breast cancer of novel PARP inhibitors (discussed later) are ongoing.

OVARIAN CANCER – CLINICAL COURSE

Numerous observational trials have consistently reported a clear survival advantage for carriers of a *BRCA* mutation, particularly those with a *BRCA2* mutation. A large pooled analysis of 26 observational studies found 5-year survival rates of 52% for *BRCA2* carriers, 44% for *BRCA1* carriers and 36% for those without a *BRCA* mutation. It is noteworthy that these studies pre-date targeted treatments, and therefore the superior survival is likely to be due to the prognostic implications of *BRCA* status and increased platinum-sensitivity [8]. Another feature is that *BRCA1/2*-deficient ovarian cancer is associated with an increased rate of visceral metastases (e.g. liver, lung splenic metastases) [9]. The subtypes of ovarian cancers associated with *BRCA1* and *BRCA2* carriers are mainly of serous or endometroid histology, with smaller numbers of mixed or clear cell subtypes. The rare subtypes, such as carcinosarcomas (mixed Müllerian tumours) appear to be under-represented in *BRCA* carriers, as are mucinous and low grade serous carcinomas.

Chemotherapy

The standard systemic treatment for epithelial ovarian cancer is platinum-based chemotherapy. First-line therapy is usually a combination of carboplatin and paclitaxel in addition to maximal cytoreductive surgery. Despite advances in surgery and systemic therapy, the majority of patients eventually relapse. Systemic options at this stage are guided by the time from last platinum – 'the platinum-free interval'. Options include platinum-based regimens, e.g. carboplatin in combination with either paclitaxel, gemcitabine, liposomal doxorubicin or as a single agent.

There has been extensive pre-clinical work performed on the mechanism of action of chemotherapeutic agents and it is recognised that an intact *BRCA* protein function may be important for the repair of cells following certain chemotherapy agents; conversely, intact *BRCA* function is necessary for some chemotherapy agents to be most effective. In support of these findings, there are several lines of clinical evidence that suggest clinical response to chemotherapy in *BRCA*-associated ovarian cancers differs from non-carriers. A retrospective study compared 22 ovarian cancer patients with germline *BRCA1* or *BRCA2* mutations to 44 nonhereditary matched control patients all of whom received primary platinum-based chemotherapy. Women with *BRCA* mutations had greater overall survival than controls (95% versus 59%, $P = 0.002$), increased complete response rates to first-line treatment (81.8% versus 43.2%, $P = 0.004$), and higher response rates to second and third line chemotherapy (second line 91.7% versus 40.9%, $P = 0.004$; third line (100% versus 14.3%, $P = 0.005$) [10]. There are preclinical data suggesting that *BRCA*-mutated ovarian cancers are relatively insensitive to microtubule-stabilising agents including paclitaxel. However, a small clinical retrospective series of 26 patients treated with single agent paclitaxel suggests that this is an active agent in *BRCA*-mutated recurrent ovarian cancer [11]. In addition, *BRCA* mutation carriers appear to have a greater sensitivity to liposomal doxorubicin.

The knowledge of mutation status can therefore be important in the selection of chemotherapy agents.

Poly (ADP-ribose) polymerase inhibitors

A major advance in systemic treatment for ovarian cancer has been the development of poly ADP-ribose polymerase (PARP) inhibitors (**Figure 8.3**). This class of drugs exploits

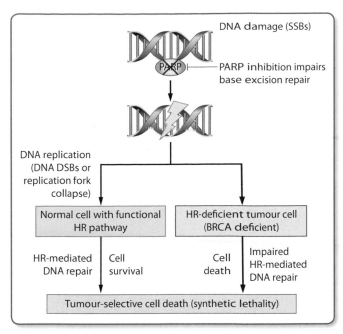

DNA damage (SSBs)

PARP inhibition impairs base excision repair

DNA replication (DNA DSBs or replication fork collapse)

Normal cell with functional HR pathway

HR-deficient tumour cell (BRCA deficient)

HR-mediated DNA repair | Cell survival

Cell death | Impaired HR-mediated DNA repair

Tumour-selective cell death (synthetic lethality)

Figure 8.3 In the presence of PARP inhibition, BRCA deficient tumour cells are unable to repair DNA damage and undergo cell death. Normal cells retain BRCA function and are able to repair DNA damage through the homologous repair (HR) pathway. With permission from Banerjee S, Kaye SB, Ashworth A. Making the best of PARP inhibitors in ovarian cancer. Nat Rev Clin Oncol 2010;7:508-519.

the concept of 'synthetic lethality' whereby a mutation in either of two genes individually has no effect, but a combination of the mutations leads to death. A drug that targets only *BRCA*-deficient tumour cells should selectively kill tumour cells while sparing non-cancer cells, which retain normal expression of *BRCA* proteins. In principle, this selectivity has the potential for a large therapeutic window. This led to the development of targeting *PARP*, a nuclear enzyme essential for the repair of single-stranded DNA breaks (SSBs) in the base excision repair (BER) pathway. The inhibition of this repair causes accumulation of SSBs and can lead to formation of double-stranded DNA breaks and collapse of the replication fork. In normal cells with intact *BRCA* protein function, the DNA lesions generated can be repaired. However, in *BRCA*-defective cancer cells, this is not possible leading to selective cell death [12]. This theory was confirmed in a Phase I proof of concept trial of the PARP inhibitor, olaparib, in a population enriched for *BRCA* mutation carriers [13].

There are several PARP inhibitors that have now shown promising activity in ovarian cancer. Of these, olaparib, is the most developed agent and has demonstrated objective clinically meaningful response rates [33% response evaluation criteria in solid tumours (RECIST) response rate at 400 mg twice daily] in heavily pretreated *BRCA* carriers with ovarian cancer in phase II trials. A wider application of PARP inhibitors was hypothesised in view of the fact that up to 50% of high-grade serous, sporadic ovarian cancers are associated with defective homologous recombination repair pathways (including *BRCA* methylation and somatic *BRCA* mutations) and therefore potentially susceptible to PARP inhibition [14]. Other germline mutations in genes including *RAD51C*, *RAD51D* and *BRIP1*, have been associated with an increased susceptibility to ovarian cancer. There is pre-clinical evidence that *RAD51D* deficient tumour cells similarly exhibit in-vitro sensitivity to PARP inhibitors, although this is yet to be tested in *RAD51C* and *BRIP1* deficient models [15]. Efficacy was shown in a Phase II study of olaparib in sporadic ovarian cancer with a response rate of 50%. This was a double-blind, placebo-controlled randomised phase II study in platinum-sensitive, recurrent, high-grade serous ovarian cancer patients who were randomised to either olaparib or placebo maintenance therapy following a response to their most recent platinum chemotherapy. The progression-free survival (PFS) (according to RECIST criteria), was almost doubled with olaparib compared to the placebo arm (median, 8.4 months versus 4.8 months; HR 0.35, P <0.001). Preliminary analysis indicate that the benefit of olaparib maintenance therapy, at least in terms of PFS, was larger in known $BRCA$ germline mutation carriers (PFS HR 0.18 (BRCA) versus 0.53 (wild-type) [16]. Other PARP inhibitors in development include rucaparib, veliparib, niraparib and BMN-673. A number of phase III studies of PARP inhibitors as maintenance therapy are planned.

PARP inhibitors as monotherapy are generally well tolerated with toxicities mainly limited to mild myelosuppression, nausea and fatigue. There have been attempts to combine PARP inhibitors with chemotherapy. However, increased myelosuppression with combinations is a limitation. Other combination strategies under investigation are PARP inhibitors with PI3K inhibitors or antiangiogenic agents. Mechanisms of resistance to PARP inhibitors are being studied and include acquired reversion of the $BRCA$ mutation.

Predictive testing and management of asymptomatic carriers

Once a mutation has been identified in an individual, predictive testing can be performed on those at risk of having inherited the mutation. It is usually clear whether the mutation is likely to have been inherited from the maternal or paternal lineage from the family history, but sometimes it may be useful to test parents (if still alive) if there is no clear history of $BRCA$-associated cancers. It is extremely rare to find de-novo (new, rather than inherited from a parent) germline mutations in the $BRCA1$ and $BRCA2$ genes. The identification of those carrying a $BRCA$ mutation before they are diagnosed with cancer allows the carriers to receive appropriate screening, and consider risk reduction strategies. It also allows suitable discussion of other issues such as contraceptive choice and pregnancy.

Screening

MRI breast imaging

The use of mammographic screening for breast cancer in women between the ages of 50 years, and 70 years has been shown to reduce breast cancer mortality by up to 25%. However, mammographic screening below this age is less effective, due to the denser breasts of pre-menopausal women. The early trials have also suggested lower detection rates of breast cancer amongst $BRCA$ carriers undergoing mammography, possibly due to innate histopathological differences and potential increased rate of growth. This led to the investigation of screening with magnetic resonance imaging (MRI), which was already being used as a diagnostic tool in breast cancer. This had the advantages that the image quality is independent of breast density, and does not have the radiation dose of mammograms. However, MRI is much more expensive than a mammogram, and the image quality can be influenced by the menstrual cycle. Overall, MRI is significantly more sensitive than mammograms (40% versus 71%) and particularly so for detection of invasive breast cancer (33% versus 79.5%). MRI is less specific than mammograms, with more women requiring additional tests or short-term follow-up [17].

Ovarian screening

To date, multiple trials have investigated the role of screening to detect ovarian cancer at an earlier stage in both general and high-risk populations. These have generally focused on ultrasound scan (abdominal or transvaginal), with or without CA125 measurement. To date, none of these trials have demonstrated ovarian screening to be effective, although the full results of a familial ovarian cancer study (UK-FOCCS) are still awaited. The examination of pathology specimens from risk-reducing salpingo-oophorectomy (RRSO) has identified pre-malignant intratubal lesions, and early invasive tubal cancers. These lesions have led to the suggestion that ovarian malignancy may originate in the fallopian tube, rather than the ovary in *BRCA* carriers (and possibly non-carriers). The presence of similar pre-malignant lesions in the ovary has not been identified. This may partly explain why ovarian screening has not been effective, as cells may spread directly from the fallopian tube into the peritoneal cavity, without an enlarged/abnormal appearing ovary on ultrasound.

Chemoprevention

There has been considerable interest in risk reduction strategies other than prophylactic surgery for unaffected women who carry a *BRCA* mutation. These have largely focused on the use of selective oestrogen receptor modulators (SERM), tamoxifen and raloxifene, although other antioestrogen agents such as aromatase inhibitors have also been investigated.

Risk-reducing salpingo-oophorectomy

The use of RRSO has been shown to significantly reduce the risk of ovarian cancer, although women retain a small risk of primary peritoneal cancer. A meta-analysis of the six main trials assessing the effect of RRSO showed an overall HR of 0.21 (risk reduction of 79%), but it should be noted that only 1 trial assessed *BRCA1* carriers alone, and none of the trials assessed *BRCA2* carriers alone. RRSO also reduces the risk of primary breast cancer (RR 0.36–0.63), with higher risk reduction rates in women who have surgery while premenopausal [18]. RRSO rates vary by country, but overall rates of uptake are increasing, and remain higher than rates of prophylactic bilateral mastectomy. The uptake rates tend to be higher in women who have had children, and those with a family history of ovarian cancer. There is some recent evidence that bilateral salpingectomy may be effective, allowing women to delay oophorectomy, and avoid many of the negative symptoms resulting from RRSO. However, more evidence is required before the full beneficial effect of this approach is clear, to determine which patients would benefit most from this approach.

Risk reducing bilateral mastectomy

The use of risk reducing bilateral mastectomy (RRBM) to reduce breast cancer risk in women with a strong family history was shown to be effective even before the discovery of the *BRCA1* and *BRCA2* genes. Subsequent studies focused on the risk reduction in unaffected women found to carry a mutation and who chose to undergo either RRBM or continue regular surveillance. These observational studies showed those who underwent RRBM had up to a 90% reduction in subsequent breast cancer risk, although the follow-up was limited [19]. The PROSE study also showed a 95% breast cancer risk reduction in carriers who had undergone both RRBM and RRSO. Despite these high rates of risk reduction, RRBM uptake remains lower than RRSO. This may be due to the more extensive surgery, and perceived cosmetic effect, as the more widespread availability of reconstructive surgery has coincided with higher rates of RRBM.

Risk reducing surgery in carriers with cancer

BRCA carriers who have already been diagnosed with cancer may still benefit from risk reducing surgery, as their risk of developing subsequent cancers is dependent on the prognosis from their initial cancer. The majority of women with breast cancer will be treated with curative intent, and may be expected to live for many more years, during which time they are at risk of developing a contralateral breast cancer (40% 10-year actuarial risk), or ovarian cancer. The risk is higher in those diagnosed with their first cancer before 40 years of age, with a 25-year risk of up to 63% of a subsequent breast cancer. These women would gain equivalent benefit from undergoing a RRSO or RRM as non-carriers. The carriers who initially develop ovarian cancer may also benefit from RRBM if they have early stage ovarian cancer, but the majority will have advanced disease at diagnosis. These women have a limited prognosis from their ovarian cancer, and gain no survival advantage from undergoing RRBM.

Pregnancy

The evidence for the effect of pregnancy and parity on the risk of breast and ovarian cancer in carriers of a BRCA mutation has been conflicting, with multiple studies showing both an increased risk and decreased risk of either cancer with BRCA1 carriers. The data for BRCA2 carriers is sparse, but overall suggest pregnancy and parity may increase the risk of breast and ovarian cancer compared with the risk for nulliparous women.

Hormone replacement treatment

For pre-menopausal women who have undergone RRSO, there was no difference in breast cancer risk reduction if hormone replacement treatment (HRT) was used until age 50 years in the prospective PROSE study. There is insufficient data on the use of HRT beyond age 50 years (i.e. beyond the age at which women would be expected to enter menopause) to recommend it currently. There is no evidence of an increased risk of primary peritoneal cancer in women given short-term HRT following RRSO. For carriers who have not undergone risk-reducing surgery, HRT may increase the risk of subsequent breast cancer development, particularly in BRCA2 carriers, who are more likely to develop hormone positive breast tumours.

Combined oral contraceptive pill

The use of the combined oral contraceptive pill (COC) has been shown to protect against ovarian cancer in BRCA carriers, but the extent of protection is influenced by length of use. In general, there appears to be ~50% risk reduction for users of the COC, but the effect on breast cancer risk is still unclear. It may be slightly increased, particularly with prolonged use. This potential risk has prevented widespread recommendation of COC as a chemopreventative agent.

Preimplantation genetic diagnosis

BRCA1 or BRCA2 mutation carriers have a 50% chance of each child inheriting the BRCA mutation. To eliminate this, some carriers may choose to consider pre-implantation genetic diagnosis (PGD). PGD is performed as part of a cycle of IVF with the embryos tested at day 3, by removing 1 or 2 cells, and screening for the familial *BRCA* mutation. The embryos that test negative for the mutation can be transferred, eliminating the risk of a child carrying the mutation. This approach is useful for those who are concerned about passing on the increased risk of breast and ovarian cancer, however uptake has been limited. There has been reluctance from some carriers to select against embryos for an adult-onset condition, when risk-reduction options are available.

Endometrial cancer

The association of endometrial cancer risk with *BRCA* mutation status is controversial. An increased risk of endometrial cancer has been demonstrated in *BRCA* carriers, but it has been difficult to differentiate whether this is a direct increased susceptibility or a consequence of tamoxifen usage in *BRCA* carriers with a history of breast cancer.

A high incidence of *BRCA1* and *BRCA2* mutations in Jewish women with serous papillary endometrial cancer has been shown in two studies, although this has not been clearly documented in non-Jewish cohorts. This histological subtype of endometrial cancer represents approximately 10% of endometrial cancer, and is characterised by a more aggressive clinical behaviour than the common endometroid subtype of endometrial cancer. *BRCA* mutation rates of 2–9% have been reported in patients with endometrial serous papillary cancer, most of who have concurrent breast cancer [20. These rates are higher than the population mutation rates of 0.2% but may be influenced by tamoxifen use, which is associated with endometrial hyperplasia, polyps and endometrial cancer.

CONCLUSION

BRCA1 and *BRCA2* mutations are reported in approximately 10% of ovarian cancer regardless of family history. More widespread *BRCA* testing for ovarian cancer patients is warranted. In addition to the importance for family members, this knowledge is likely to influence an individual patient's treatment options. PARP inhibitors are showing exceptional promise for patients with *BRCA*-associated ovarian cancer and the effects may extend to non-germline *BRCA* mutation associated ovarian cancer.

Key points for clinical practice

- Germline *BRCA* mutations are present in about 10% of women with epithelial ovarian cancers.
- A family history is not present in up to 50% of women with ovarian cancer who carry a *BRCA* mutation.
- Women with ovarian cancer who carry a *BRCA* mutation tend to have a different clinical course compared to non-carriers (younger age at diagnosis, increased sensitivity to platinum, visceral metastases, high grade serous histology).
- Bilateral salpingo-oophorectomy significantly reduces the risk of both breast and ovarian cancer in unaffected carriers of a *BRCA* mutation.
- PARP inhibitors have shown encouraging results in phase II studies of *BRCA*-associated ovarian cancer.
- Phase III studies of PARP inhibitors as maintenance therapy in ovarian cancer are planned.

REFERENCES

1. Hall JM, Lee MK, Newman B, et al. Linkage of early-onset familial breast cancer to chromosome 17q21. Science 1990; 250:1684–1689.
2. Narod SA, Feunteun J, Lynch HT, et al. Familial breast-ovarian cancer locus on chromosome 17q12-q23. Lancet 1991; 338:82–83.
3. Wooster R, Bignell G, Lancaster J, et al. Identification of the breast cancer susceptibility gene BRCA2. Nature 1995; 378:789–792.
4. Gayther SA, Mangion J, Russell P, et al. Variation of risks of breast and ovarian cancer associated with different germline mutations of the BRCA2 gene. Nat Genet 1997; 15:103–105.
5. Tonin P, Weber B, Offit K, et al. Frequency of recurrent BRCA1 and BRCA2 mutations in Ashkenazi Jewish breast cancer families. Nat Med 1996; 2:1179–1183.
6. Antoniou AC, Hardy R, Walker L, et al. Predicting the likelihood of carrying a BRCA1 or BRCA2 mutation: validation of BOADICEA, BRCAPRO, IBIS, Myriad and the Manchester scoring system using data from UK genetics clinics. J Med Genet 2008; 45:425–431.
7. Alsop K, Fereday S, Meldrum C, et al. BRCA mutation frequency and patterns of treatment response in BRCA mutation-positive women with ovarian cancer: a report from the Australian Ovarian Cancer Study Group. J Clin Oncol 2012; 30:2654–2663.
8. Bolton KL, Chenevix-Trench G, Goh C, et al. Association between BRCA1 and BRCA2 mutations and survival in women with invasive epithelial ovarian cancer. JAMA 2012; 307:382–390.
9. Gourley C, Michie CO, Roxburgh P, et al. Increased incidence of visceral metastases in scottish patients with BRCA1/2-defective ovarian cancer: An extension of the ovarian BRCAness Phenotype. J Clin Oncol 2010; 28:2505–2511.
10. Tan DSP, Rothermundt C, Thomas K, et al. 'BRCAness' syndrome in ovarian cancer: Control study describing the clinical features and outcome of patients with epithelial ovarian cancer associated with BRCA1 and BRCA2 mutations. J Clin Oncol 2008; 26:5530–5536.
11. Tan DS, Yap TA, Hutka M, et al. Implications of BRCA1 and BRCA2 mutations for the efficacy of paclitaxel monotherapy in advanced ovarian cancer. Eur J Cancer 2013; 49:1246–1253.
12. Farmer H, McCabe N, Lord CJ, et al. Targeting the DNA repair defect in BRCA mutant cells as a therapeutic strategy. Nature 2005; 434:917–921.
13. Fong PC, Boss DS, Yap TA, et al. Inhibition of poly(ADP-ribose) polymerase in tumors from BRCA mutation carriers. N Engl J Med 2009; 361:123–134.
14. Banerjee S, Kaye S. PARP inhibitors in BRCA gene-mutated ovarian cancer and beyond. Curr Oncol Rep. 2011; 13:442–449.
15. Loveday C, Turnbull C, Ramsay E, et al. Germline mutations in RAD51D confer susceptibility to ovarian cancer. Nat Genet 2011; 43:879–884.
16. Ledermann J, Harter P, Gourley C, et al. Olaparib maintenance therapy in platinum-sensitive relapsed ovarian cancer. N Engl J Med 2012; 366:1382–1392.
17. Kriege M, Brekelmans CT, Boetes C, et al. Efficacy of MRI and mammography for breast-cancer screening in women with a familial or genetic predisposition. N Engl J Med 2004; 351:427–437.
18. Rebbeck TR, Kauff ND, Domchek SM. Meta-analysis of risk reduction estimates associated with risk-reducing salpingo-oophorectomy in BRCA1 or BRCA2 mutation carriers. J Natl Cancer Inst 2009; 101:80–87.
19. Rebbeck TR, Friebel T, Lynch HT, et al. Bilateral prophylactic mastectomy reduces breast cancer risk in BRCA1 and BRCA2 mutation carriers: the PROSE study Group. J Clin Oncol 2004; 22:1055–1062.
20. Segev Y, Iqbal J, Lubinski J, et al. The incidence of endometrial cancer in women with BRCA1 and BRCA2 mutations: An international prospective cohort study. Gynecol Oncol 2013; 130:127–131.

Chapter 9

Management of pregnancy following in vitro fertilisation with egg donation

Surabhi Nanda, Catherine Nelson-Piercy

INTRODUCTION

In vitro fertilisation (IVF) with egg donation (ED) is now an established technique in assisted reproduction. Since its introduction in the early 1980s, this technique now accounts for over 4% of all assisted reproductive technology (ART) [1, 2]. The average age of first conception in western society is rising. In 2009, women over 35 accounted for nearly 53% of all ART. The European Society of Human Reproduction and Embryology (ESHRE) in its 13th annual report on European data on noted an increase in ED, with nearly 8000 more cycles than the previous report [2]. IVF with ED has better success rates that IVF alone in women with poor or diminishing ovarian reserve (Table 9.1).

IVF is a known independent risk factor for various antenatal and perinatal complications. In the seventh report of the confidential enquiries into maternal deaths in the United Kingdom, 12 women were known to have undergone IVF, three resulting in a multiple pregnancy. The most frequent direct cause of death was ovarian hyperstimulation syndrome (OHSS) followed by sepsis, venous thromboembolism and bleeding, not related to IVF. From a reanalysis of data by the human fertilisation and embryology authority (HFEA), the estimated rate of maternal death was calculated to be 12 per 100,000 ART cycles [3]. No separate mortality data are currently available for IVF with ED. Successful

Table 9.1 Pregnancy and delivery rates per transfer of embryo [2]		
Technique	Pregnancy/transfer (%)	Delivery/transfer (%)
In vitro fertilisation	32.9	23
Intracytoplasmic sperm injection	32.0	21.5
Egg donation	45.7	30.2

Surabhi Nanda MRCOG, St Thomas' Hospital, London, UK. Email: surabhi.nanda@kcl.ac.uk.

Catherine Nelson-Piercy MA FRCP FRCOG, St Thomas' Hospital, London, UK.
Email: catherine.nelson-piercy@gstt.nhs.uk (for correspondence)

pregnancy with IVF with ED is an immune paradox as the fetal genome is completely different to the mother's. Evidence on IVF with ED suggests that these pregnancies are at a higher risk compared to natural conception or pregnancies with IVF alone [4–6]. It is postulated that some of the adverse outcomes in IVF with ED pregnancies are due to the allogenic nature of the fetus [7].

Although ED was initially offered for women with premature ovarian failure, it has been extended to assist couples to overcome infertility from multiple factors, e.g. diminished ovarian reserve, recurrent implantation failure, recurrent miscarriage and various heritable genetic conditions. Good clinical practice and various medical societies suggest that there should be a comprehensive medical evaluation by a physician familiar with the risks of specific medical conditions, in particular relation to pregnancy. This should be done prior to commencing ART[8]. Women with advanced maternal age should be counselled to consider short- and long-term parenting and child-rearing issues specific to their age and the possible effects of pregnancy on their own health [9]. Pre-pregnancy counselling, especially in women with complex medical conditions plays a vital role in planning what could be a high-risk pregnancy and optimising the chances of a favourable outcome, both for the mother and the fetus/es.

IN VITRO FERTILISATION WITH EGG DONATION – OVERVIEW OF TECHNIQUE

Egg donation involves use of a donor oocyte obtained from a fresh IVF cycle from a suitable screened donor, which is fertilised with the recipient's partner's sperm. The fertilised embryo is transferred to the uterus of the recipient after treatment to produce a receptive secretory evolution. Unfertilised mature oocytes are obtained from a donor who should be younger than 37 years old, healthy and preferably of known fertility. A routine IVF cycle is then performed, and depending on the sperm parameters of the male partner of the recipient, the eggs are fertilised either routinely or with intracytoplasmic sperm injection (ICSI). The resultant embryos can be replaced fresh or in a frozen cycle. If the recipient's menstrual cycle is regular the embryos can be replaced in a natural cycle. However in peri- or postmenopausal women, the endometrium of the recipient must be primed with oestrogen and progesterone before transfer of the embryos, and hormonal supplementation must be maintained for at least 10 weeks. The quality of the embryos depends on the donor egg and the partner's sperm parameters. The number of embryos transferred is decided based on the age of the donor, not the age of the recipient and as such with advanced donor age, a single embryo transfer is strongly recommended in order to minimise the risk of multiple pregnancy [8].

COMMON INDICATIONS FOR IN VITRO FERTILISATION WITH EGG DONATION

Initially offered to women with premature ovarian failure, the technique of ED is now used to achieve pregnancy for a variety of conditions (Table 9.2) [10–15, 40]. There are extensive data on successful ED pregnancies in Turner's syndrome and Turner's mosaics, although some studies quote a higher miscarriage rate compared to IVF-ED for other indications

Table 9.2 Indications for IVF with egg donation [10–15, 40]

Women with no/minimal ovarian reserve
1. Advanced maternal age (≥43 years)
2. Premature ovarian failure
   a. Genetic causes
      i. Chromosomal
         1. Turner's syndrome and Turner's mosaics
         2. Pure gonadal dysgenesis/Swyer's syndrome
         3. Fragile X
         4. Familial
      ii. Metabolic
         1. 17 α-hydroxylase deficiency
         2. Galactosaemia
         3. Myotonic dystrophy
      iii. Immunological
         1. Di George syndrome
         2. Ataxia telangiectasia
         3. Mucocutaneous fungal infections
   b. Autoimmune disease, commonly
      i. Hypothyroidism
      ii. Diabetes
      iii. Addison's
      iv. Autoimmune oophoritis
   c. Environmental
   d. Infections (e.g. mumps)
   e. Iatrogenic
      i. Surgical
      ii. Chemotherapy [e.g. alkylating agents–cyclophosphamide, nitrosoureas, chlorambucil, melphalan, busulfan; vinca alkaloids (vinblastine); platinum agents–cisplatin; antimetabolites (cytarabine)]
         1. Childhood or young adulthood cancers
         2. Treatment for autoimmune conditions
      iii. Irradiation
   f. Idiopathic
3. Resistant ovary/Savage syndrome

Women with normal ovarian reserve
1. Repeated failed attempts at IVF/poor responders
   a. Failure to respond to ovarian stimulation regimens
   b. Repeated failed egg collection or inaccessible ovaries,e.g. because of adhesions
   c. Failure of fertilisation of apparently normal oocytes and spermatozoa
   d. Failed implantation of embryos with apparently normal uterus
2. Genetic conditions
   a. Autosomal dominant conditions (affecting the recipient)
   b. Both partners carrier of an autosomal recessive condition (and donor insemination not acceptable or feasible)
   c. Some X-linked disorders
   d. Family history of a genetic condition and where carrier status cannot be determined or gene not known (e.g. familial recurrent hydatidiform molar pregnancy)
   e. Unexplained recurrent pregnancy losses
3. Older women with normal menstrual cycle

[14–15]. Advancing maternal age is increasingly becoming a common indication for IVF with ED. IVF units, governed by regulatory bodies like HFEA, may reserve a right to discourage ED to women after their natural menopause, especially those with other medical comorbidities. Poor responders to traditional IVF techniques or women who have suffered recurrent pregnancy losses due to aneuploidies or other unexplained causes may also be suitable candidates for IVF with ED. It is unclear, however, whether women presenting with antiphospholipid syndrome or inherited thrombophilia would benefit from ED, and current practice is to offer ED in these women only if there are other absolute indications for ED. A woman with an autosomal dominant condition or who is a carrier of an X-linked disorder may opt for IVF with ED in order to avoid transmission of the condition to offspring. However, with advances in preimplantation genetic diagnosis and screening, these women may have an option to use their own screened oocytes or embryos for IVF. Cases of live births with embryos from donated oocytes have been reported in women who have been treated with bone marrow transplantation following total body irradiation and cyclophosphamide for leukaemia and following radical surgery (with uterine conservation) and chemotherapy for ovarian cancer [16].

SCREENING FOR ASSOCIATED MEDICAL CO-MORBIDITY PRIOR TO ART

Detailed screening recommendations for oocyte donor and recipients are outside the remit of this chapter. However, screening prior to ART presents an opportunity for comprehensive medical evaluation of the recipient. In our practice, a pre-ART consultation with an obstetric physician for those with co-morbidity to assess medical suitability for IVF is encouraged. This ensures that the ART cycle is as medically 'safe' for the recipient as possible and that she and her fertility specialist are informed of any likely complications resulting from hormonal priming or pregnancy and delivery itself. There is a recommendation that all women with premature ovarian failure should undertake an evaluation for autoimmune disorders to exclude concurrent endocrine failure [13]. Being aware of (and controlling) disease activity preconception in cases of chronic inflammatory or autoimmune disease improves the chances of a successful outcome in an IVF-ED pregnancy. For some women with severe organ impairment such as chronic kidney disease, heart failure or lung disease, pregnancy may be associated with significant risks to the woman's long-term health and, therefore, although possible may be inadvisable or IVF may be deferred, for example until after renal transplant. Such ethical dilemmas require careful counselling with the woman and her partner and multidisciplinary discussion within the assisted conception unit.

CONSIDERATIONS IN A PREGNANCY WITH IVF-ED

Age

It is well documented that advanced maternal age is associated with adverse perinatal and medical outcomes [17]. This is irrespective of the mode of conception. Advancing age also provides a platform for natural history of chronic conditions to unfold, thereby making a pregnancy even more high risk. Conditions like chronic hypertension, type 2 diabetes, cardiovascular disease and thrombosis become more prevalent with age. Older women are more likely to be obese. Certain malignancies are more common in women with delayed child bearing [18]. In addition, some women may enter their respective pregnancies having had treatment for malignancies earlier in their life and still have sequelae of treatment.

Turner's syndrome

Pregnant women with Turner's syndrome (TS) require tertiary medical and obstetric care due to increased risk for pregnancy related complications like thyroid dysfunction, obesity, diabetes, hypertension and pre-eclampsia, which occur in approximately 40% of patients with TS compared to 6–12% of the general population [19]. Severe complications include deterioration of congenital heart disease, cardiac failure, aortic dissection and sudden death. Women with TS are at increased risk of development of aortic cystic medial necrosis independent of congenital heart disease; 10% of patients with aortic dilatation, dissection, or rupture have no prior cardiac risk factors. Women with TS are at significant risk for aortopathy. Due to shorter stature, it is important to assess aortic size corrected for body surface area (aortic size index), although dissection can still occur at smaller aortic sizes in the absence of valve and arch abnormalities [20]. In a review of 101 TS pregnancies from oocyte donation programs in the United States, the risk of maternal death due to aortic dissection was estimated to be at least 2% [21]. The risk of aortic dissection is associated with factors such as congenital cardiovascular malformation (particularly bicuspid aortic valve, coarctation of the aorta and aortic root dilatation), history of lymphoedema, hypertension, obesity and multiple pregnancy [22]. Multiple embryo transfer is strongly contraindicated in women with TS [15].

Involvement of a cardiologist with expertise in adult congenital heart disease and pregnancy for pre-pregnancy risk assessment and frequent review during pregnancy is recognised as essential. Initial evaluation should include echocardiogram and MRI of cardiac anatomy and aortic dimensions, although it is unclear whether this screening will eliminate any risk as normal aortic dimensions do not exclude the risk of sudden aortic dissection. Regular pregnancy surveillance is recommended to minimise peripartum complications and decide on a mode of delivery safe for both mother and the fetus.

Complications related to assisted reproductive technology

Various ART registries suggest better pregnancy per transfer rate in IVF-ED compared to IVF with autologous eggs. There seems to be better implantation and as a result the overall miscarriage rates are slightly lower. The risk of ovarian hyperstimulation is minimised in IVF-ED as there is no superovulation of the recipient ovaries. However, there is still hormonal exposure, especially a slightly longer and cyclical oestrogen and progesterone exposure in postmenopausal women to increase the receptivity of the uterus. This needs to be considered during risk assessment of women with either a previous history or an increased risk of thromboembolism.

Psychological aspects

A recent qualitative study on the perceptions of women with advanced age in their respective pregnancies highlighted significant anxiety and psychological concerns. This was more marked in women who had other risk factors such as pregnancy complications, limited physical activity, previous poor reproductive history, and who recognised their age as a risk factor for their pregnancy [23].

PREGNANCY OUTCOMES IN PREGNANCIES WITH IVF-ED

Maternal fetal outcomes following egg donation are generally favourable and similar to results seen following conventional IVF.

The incidence of first trimester and second trimester bleeding is substantially higher when compared with standard IVF and spontaneously conceived pregnancies. This may be attributed to abnormal placentation.

The incidence of perinatal complications (intrauterine growth retardation, low birth weight, prematurity, congenital malformation) is comparable, and elevated risks (relative to the general population) are primarily related to the high incidence of multiple gestations. However, IVF-ED pregnancies have been associated with a higher incidence of pre-eclampsia and increased caesarean section rates. Pregnant recipients above the age of 40 years are at an increased risk for gestational diabetes, pre-eclampsia and thrombophlebitis and above the age of 45 years they are at an increased risk of hypertension, proteinuria, premature rupture of membranes, second- and third-trimester haemorrhage, preterm delivery and lower mean infant birth weights [7]. One study that corrected for maternal age and multiple gestation concluded that women who conceived with donor oocytes remain at high risk for preterm labour, pre-eclampsia and protracted labour, requiring caesarean section delivery [24]. The rate of caesarean section deliveries in ED pregnancies is increased compared with spontaneous conceptions [7]. Much of this increase may be related to obstetrician decision to perform elective caesarean sections in view of the IVF-ED and/or increased maternal age, rather than for specific obstetric or medical indications.

A recent retrospective cohort study looking at pregnancy outcomes in IVF-ED pregnancies in women over 43 years showed that such pregnancies have a significantly higher risk of pre-eclampsia compared with pregnant women without IVF [adjusted OR 3.3 (1.2–8.9)]. This increase may be explained by the increased 'immunological load' of an embro/s where all (as opposed to 50%) of genetic material in the uteroplacental unit is foreign to the mother. The rate of twin pregnancy was significantly higher in women with IVF and oocyte donation (39.4 versus 15.0% with IVF only and 2.5% without IVF, $P < 0.001$). Twin pregnancy was significantly associated with increased risk of preterm delivery [adjusted OR 8.9 (4.0–19.9)] and PPH [adjusted OR 3.5 (1.3–9.5)] [25]. A recent Danish national cohort study of 375 children born following IVF-ED showed a higher incidence of preterm birth and low birth weight compared to those born after spontaneous conception, but attributed this largely to pre-eclampsia in the ED group [26]. Two other large American studies comparing IVF-ED with routine IVF showed a significant increase in low birth weight and preterm births. However, in both these studies there was no correction for pre-eclampsia [26, 27]. Early growth and development of children born to recipients has only been sporadically studied but appears similar to the background population [28].

There are limited data available on outcome of pregnancies in IVF-ED stratified for the reason for ED (apart from advanced maternal age). In addition, it is possible that the fertility status of the egg donor may have an impact on the overall pregnancy outcome. However, in the Danish cohort, pregnancy outcomes from oocytes from donors undergoing fertility treatment (egg sharing) and fertile or parous donors were similar [25].

MANAGEMENT OF PREGNANCY WITH ED

Pre-pregnancy

The care of a woman with IVF-ED should commence before the ART cycle. Routine counselling should include advice regarding commencing folic acid at least 3 months prior to planned pregnancy (5 mg depending on the concurrent medical condition), cessation of smoking, reduction or cessation of alcohol. There should be a discussion concerning medications that are safe periconceptionally and in pregnancy [30]. These women should be counselled about the risk of multiple pregnancies, hypertensive disorders in pregnancy and preterm labour.

Pre-pregnancy counselling and a medical evaluation enable prepregnancy risk assessment of these women. A clinician should perform a comprehensive medical examination including cardiovascular (and other endocrine system examination where indicated). Information regarding prepregnancy blood pressure and/or proteinuria is vital due to the increased risk of developing pre-eclampsia. Routine tests like rhesus genotyping, haemoglobinopathy screening, virology screen, cervical smear should be performed as a part of pre-ART investigations.

Single embryo transfer

The majority of adverse pregnancy outcomes in IVF-ED pregnancies are either linked to pre-eclampsia or to multiple gestations. Even with the transfer of only two cleavage-stage embryos derived from donor oocytes, multiple gestation rates of near 40% can be expected [31] and may be greater than 50% with transfer of two blastocyst-stage embryos [32]. The recent American Society of Reproductive Medicine guidelines for selective single embryo transfer (SET) recommend IVF with ED as having one of the best prognoses with SET [33]. This is further advisable particularly in women with other medical co-morbidities, where a multiple pregnancy may worsen both maternal and fetal outcomes.

Early pregnancy

A pregnancy conceived with IVF-ED, irrespective of the indication for ED, should be considered a high-risk pregnancy. This would warrant an early obstetric antenatal appointment. The first appointment is an opportunity to re-iterate the maternal fetal risks, to ensure that ongoing medication is safe in pregnancy and to devise and agree an antenatal schedule.

An early pregnancy scan should be arranged (if not already done via the IVF unit) to assess the viability and the number of fetuses. This is an optimal time to establish chorionicity in a multiple pregnancy.

Once a viable pregnancy is confirmed, 75 mg of low dose aspirin is recommended until at least 36 weeks' gestation. There is evidence from various studies that aspirin started at ≤16 weeks is associated with a significant reduction in severe pre-eclampsia (relative risk: 0.22, 95% CI: 0.08–0.57) [34]. Although National Institute for Clinical Excellence (NICE) recommends starting low dose aspirin from 12 weeks, this is because there are few robust safety data for use in the first trimester [35]. Many clinicians including the authors feel that starting aspirin as soon as possible may be beneficial and is not associated with increased risks.

First trimester

Following IVF, the majority of women receive progesterone supplementation, which can be discontinued at the end of first trimester. Some IVF units would commence low molecular weight heparin (LMWH) as an adjuvant therapy, particularly if there has been a history of recurrent miscarriage or poor response to IVF. Risk assessment for venous thromboembolism (VTE) should be undertaken early in pregnancy [36]. If there is no absolute indication for thromboprophylaxis, LMWH should be discontinued at the end of the first trimester. However, many women undergoing IVF-ED are at intermediate or high risk for venous thromboembolism on the basis of their age, medical comorbidity, IVF and multiple pregnancy. Therefore, an individual VTE risk assessment is vital to decide on antenatal thromboprophylaxis and/or duration of postnatal thromboprophylaxis [36].

ART in itself is a risk factor for VTE. However, this is on the basis of the risk of OHSS. As women undergoing IVF-ED have no superovulation, and essentially get a short cycle of hormonal treatment, it is the risk for VTE in IVF-ED based solely on ART as a risk factor is the same as for women undergoing routine IVF.

If additional investigations were not performed earlier, e.g. baseline blood tests (where indicated – FBC, U&E, LFT, TFT, CRP, ESR or ANA, complements depending on any underlying disease) this is a good time to assess them. A baseline echocardiogram for women with TS or structural heart disease can be performed. Cardiac MRI, if indicated, to rule out an aneurysm especially for women with repaired aortopathies (TS or Turner's mosaics) should be delayed until after the first trimester.

11–13 week scan (combined screening)

The fetal medicine foundation algorithm for first trimester aneuploidy screening provides a background risk for trisomy 21, 13 and 18 based on the maternal age. The patient specific risk is calculated based on a multiple risk factor model which incorporates nuchal translucency, additional markers (where available) including nasal bone, ductus venosus flow and tricuspid regurgitation, maternal serum β-human chorionic gonadotrophin and placental associated plasma protein-A, in addition to the age of the mother (in this case donor), ethnicity and other factors like smoking or type 1 diabetes. It is important to incorporate the ART details – donor age, and the day of transfer for precise risk assessment [37]. Women with TS are at high risk of aneuploid pregnancies, in particular trisomy 21 [19]. This would be considered in the risk algorithm for trisomy screening at 11–13 weeks in a routine IVF or a spontaneous pregnancy. However, this would be disregarded in an IVF-ED pregnancy, because of different maternal genetic material. The National Institute for Clinical Excellence recommends dating the pregnancy based on the crown rump length measurement at the 11–13 weeks scan [38]. The exception to the rule is a pregnancy conceived following any form of ART.

Second trimester

18–20 week scan (anomaly)

There is a paucity of larger studies and long-term follow-up data on the risk of congenital malformations in pregnancies conceived with ED compared to other ART techniques. However, data on ART suggest an increased risk of congenital malformations in pregnancies with IVF compared to spontaneous conception. The risk is further increased in IVF with ICSI. Maternal age and quality of eggs would not be a confounding factor in IVF-ED; however, multiple pregnancy remains a major risk factor for congenital malformations in this group [39].

The NHS anomaly screening program recommends a detailed structural anomaly scan for all pregnancies between 18+0 to 20+6 weeks' gestation. In our practice, we recommend uterine artery Doppler studies in addition to the routine anomaly scan. A high resistance utero-placental circulation as reflected by a uterine artery pulsatility index greater than the 95th centile would warrant additional surveillance for pre-eclampsia and growth restriction.

There are no additional indication for specialist fetal echocardiography. The routine indications such as personal or first-degree relative history of cardiac abnormality, maternal Ro/La antibodies, and use of antiepileptic drugs or monochorionic twin pregnancies would also apply for IVF-ED conceptions.

Third trimester

If the woman is screen positive for risk of pre-eclampsia or IUGR (based on the biophysical or biochemical markers of abnormal placentation as reflected in abnormal utero-placental blood flow at anomaly scan and maternal serum PAPP-A below the 5th centile at combined screening), additional growth scans are arranged 4 weekly. We recommend fortnightly antenatal checks in such women till 32–34 weeks and then at least weekly. Additional growth scans for fetal surveillance are recommended in twin pregnancy (2–3 weekly – monochorionic or 4 weekly – dichorionic) or with a diagnosis of pre-eclampsia (2 weekly, usually) or due to underlying medical co-morbidity [e.g. chronic hypertension, maternal diabetes, chronic kidney disease, antiphospholipid syndrome (APS) or systemic lupus erythematosus (SLE)].

Timing and mode of delivery is based on whether there is evidence of any underlying maternal or fetal compromise or pregnancy complications. IVF-ED alone is not an indication for an earlier delivery, although maternal anxiety can occasionally lead to requests for elective caesarean sections or induction of labour before 40 weeks. There is evidence that women with advanced maternal age, irrespective of parity have higher perinatal complications like stillbirth, emergency caesarean section, and postpartum haemorrhage [17]. Consequently, there is a practice in some units to offer induction of labour around 38–39 weeks for such women.

If the pregnancy has remained uncomplicated, IVF-ED alone is not a contraindication for delivery in a midwifery led birthing unit. This may, however, not be practical in standalone midwifery units with no on-site obstetric support. This may be an opportunity to de-medicalise the pregnancy, where appropriate. In our unit, we recommend a prelabour agreement with the obstetrician and lead midwifery staff, if the woman intends to deliver in a low-risk birth setting. Such a discussion includes a detailed plan for potential obstetric input or indications for transfer to the high-risk birth centre.

Women with TS deserve a special mention. In the presence of cardiovascular compromise like significant coarctation of aorta or aortic root dilatation, planned caesarean section is likely to be the preferred option for delivery

Postnatal

The duration of postnatal thromboprophylaxis is decided based on the mode of delivery and ongoing risk factors for venous thromboembolism. If there were medical risk factors which were directly or indirectly associated with the indication for ED, or if there were specific pregnancy associated conditions like early onset pre-eclampsia, severe obstetric cholestasis or extreme prematurity, a follow-up is recommended in an obstetric medicine/high-risk obstetric clinic around 6–8 weeks postpartum. This is an appropriate time to discuss contraception. Progesterone based preparations are usually recommended especially when oestrogen containing preparations are contraindicated, e.g. in older women, women with previous thromboembolism, or conditions like obstetric cholestasis.

Pregnancies with IVF-ED, as discussed above, need the input of at the very least a high-risk obstetrician or a maternal fetal medicine specialist; an obstetric physician or a physician with relevant experience and interest in dealing with medical complications of pregnancy, and specialist midwives who can offer care and psychological support to such women. There may be a combination of risk factors each of which need to be dealt individually. However, when making a care plan, a holistic multidisciplinary approach needs to be taken to ensure a successful outcome.

For example, an older primigravida with IVF-ED dichorionic diamniotic (DCDA) twin pregnancy with early onset severe obstetric cholestasis (OC) in preterm labour at 34 weeks. She had iatrogenic premature ovarian failure due to multiple cycles of chemotherapy after disseminated cancer in her 30s. Following chemotherapy she developed multiple pulmonary emboli. She was taking warfarin pre-pregnancy and switched to high prophylactic doses of low molecular weight heparin (LMWH) in the pregnancy. She was admitted in early preterm labour and needed a category two emergency caesarean section for fetal distress with postpartum haemorrhage needing packed red cells and fresh frozen plasma. She made a good recovery and was discharged back to oral anticoagulation clinic to commence warfarin on day seven.

Such a patient needed careful counselling in the first trimester regarding switching to warfarin; appropriate thromboprophylaxis; regular growth surveillance for the twin pregnancy, especially in light of her OC which needed input of the obstetric physicians as it was early onset (24 weeks), and needed titration to high doses of urosodeoxycholic acid. Haematology opinion was sought at the time of her caesarean section due to her major obstetric haemorrhage (risk factors: age, twin pregnancy, prophylactic LMWH, obstetric cholestasis).

ETHICAL ISSUES WITH EGG DONATION

Oocyte donation for women with premature ovarian failure, gonadal dysgenesis, poor oocyte quality, or diminished ovarian reserve falls into the realm of medical treatment. However, the practice is ethically problematic when oocyte or embryo donation is used as treatment for women who have experienced natural menopause. The level of maternal anxiety is high in most women with IVF-ED and many of them need extra psychosocial support. Inevitably, there is a high demand for earlier delivery or planned caesarean section. Clinicians dealing with such pregnancies often face a dilemma given the conflicts of wishing to demedicalise the pregnancy versus offering intervention where indicated.

Key points for clinical practice

- IVF-ED is a successful ART technique of choice in women with premature ovarian failure and advanced maternal age.
- Overall successful pregnancy rates in IVF-ED are better compared to IVF with autologous eggs or spontaneous conception in the selected patient groups.
- Pregnancies with IVF-ED are at risk of first- and second-trimester bleeding, pre-eclampsia, multiple gestation and increased operative delivery.
- Maternal and fetal risks in women conceiving with IVF-ED are higher when there are co-existing medical conditions.
- Pre-pregnancy counselling helps risk assessment and successful planning of pregnancies.
- Multidisciplinary and, where indicated, tertiary level of antenatal care may help reduce adverse perinatal outcomes.
- Where indicated, attempts should be made to de-medicalise the pregnancy.

REFERENCES

1. Lutjen P, Trounson A, Leeton J, et al. The establishment and maintenance of pregnancy using in vitro fertilisation and embryo donation in a patient with primary ovarian failure. Nature 1984; 307:174–175.
2. Ferraretti AP, Goossens V, Kupka M, et al. Assisted reproductive technology in Europe, 2009: results generated from European registers by ESHRE. Hum Reprod 2013; 28:2318–2331.
3. Lewis G. The confidential enquiry into maternal and child health (CEMACH). Saving Mothers' Lives: reviewing maternal deaths to make motherhood safer – 2003–2005. The seventh report on confidential enquiries into maternal deaths in the United Kingdom. London: CEMACH, 2007.
4. Sheffer-Mimouni G, Mashiach S, Dor J, et al. Factors influencing the obstetric and perinatal outcome after oocyte donation. Hum Reprod 2002; 17:2636–2640.
5. Krieg SA, Henne MB, Westphal LM. Obstetric outcomes in donor oocyte pregnancies compared with advanced maternal age in in vitro fertilization pregnancies. Fertil Steril 2008; 90:65–70.
6. Stoop D, Baumgarten M, Haentjens P, et al. Obstetric outcome in donor oocyte pregnancies: a matched-pair analysis. Reprod Biol Endocrinol 2012; 10:42.
7. Van der Hoorn ML, Lashley EE, Bianchi DW, et al. Clinical and immunologic aspects of egg donation pregnancies: a systematic review. Hum Reprod Update 2010; 16:704–712.
8. Practice Committee of American Society for Reproductive Medicine; Practice Committee of Society for Assisted Reproductive Technology. Recommendations for gamete and embryo donation: a committee opinion. Fertil Steril 2013; 99:47–62.
9. Reproductive Endocrinology and Infertility Committee; Family Physicians Advisory Committee; Maternal–Fetal Medicine Committee; Executive and Council of the Society of Obstetricians, Liu K, Case A. Advanced reproductive age and fertility. J Obstet Gynaecol Can 2011; 33:1165–1175.
10. Fisher RA, Lavery SA, Carby A, et al. What a difference an egg makes. Lancet 2011; 378:1974.
11. Abdalla HI. Ovum donation. Curr Opin Obstet Gynecol 1991; 3:674–677.
12. Coughlan C, Ledger B, Ola B. In-vitro fertilization. Obstet Gynaecol Reprod Med 2011; 21:303–310.
13. Lebovic DI, Naz R. Premature ovarian failure: think 'autoimmune disorder'. Sexual Reprod Menopause 2004; 2: 230–233.
14. Bryman I, Sylvén L, Berntorp K, et al. Pregnancy rate and outcome in Swedish women with Turner syndrome. Fertil Steril 2011; 95:2507–2510.
15. Mercadal BA, Imbert R, Demeestere I, et al. Pregnancy outcome after oocyte donation in patients with Turner's syndrome and partial X monosomy. Hum Reprod 2011; 26:2061–2068.
16. National Institute for Health and Care Excellence (NICE). Fertility: assessment and treatment of people with fertility problems. NICE clinical guideline CG156. London: NICE, 2013.
17. Kenny LC, Lavender T, McNamee R, et al. Advanced maternal age and adverse pregnancy outcome: evidence from a large contemporary cohort. PLoS One 2013; 8:e56583.
18. Nassar AH, Usta IM. Advanced maternal age. Part II: long-term consequences. Am J perinatol 2009; 26:107–112.
19. Hewitt JK, Jayasinghe Y, Amor DJ, et al. Fertility in Turner syndrome. Clin Endocrinol (Oxf) 2013; 79:606–614.
20. Matura LA, Ho VB, Rosing DR, Bondy CA. Aortic dilatation and dissection in Turner syndrome. Circulation 2007; 116:1663–1670.
21. Karnis MF, Zimon AE, Lalwani SI, et al. Risk of death in pregnancy achieved through oocyte donation in patients with Turner syndrome: a national survey. Fertil Steril 2003; 80:498–501.
22. Bondy C, Rosing D, Reindollar R. Cardiovascular risks of pregnancy in women with Turner syndrome. Fertil Steril 2009; 91:e31–32.
23. Bayrampour H, Heaman M, Duncan KA, et al. Advanced maternal age and risk perception: a qualitative study. BMC Pregnancy Childbirth 2012; 12:100.
24. Henne MB, Zhang M, Paroski S, et al. Comparison of obstetric outcomes in recipients of donor oocytes vs. women of advanced maternal age with autologous oocytes. J Reprod Med 2007; 52:585–590.
25. Le Ray C, Scherier S, Anselem O, et al. Association between oocyte donation and maternal and perinatal outcomes in women aged 43 years or older. Hum Reprod 2012; 27:896–901.
26. Malchau SS, Loft A, Larsen EC, et al. Perinatal outcomes in 375 children born after oocyte donation: a Danish national cohort study. Fertil Steril 2013; 99:1637–1643.
27. Zegers-Hochchild F, Masoli D, Schwarze JE, et al. Reproductive performance in oocyte donors and their recipients: comparative analysis from implantation to birth and lactation. Fertil Steril 2010; 93:2210–2215.
28. Gibbons WE, Cedars M, Ness RB. Toward understanding obstetrical outcome in advanced assisted reproduction: varying sperm, oocyte and uterine source and diagnosis. Fertil Steril 2011; 95:1645–1649.

29. Söderström-Anttila V, Sajaniemi N, Tiitinen A, et al. Health and development of children born after oocyte donation compared with that of those born after in-vitro fertilization, and parents' attitudes regarding secrecy. Hum Reprod 1998; 13:2009–2015.
30. Seshadri S, Oakeshott P, Nelson-Piercy C, et al. Prepregnancy care. BMJ. 2012; 344:e3467.
31. Adashi EY, Barri PN, Berkowitz R, et al. Infertility therapy-associated multiple pregnancies (births): an ongoing epidemic. Reprod Biomed Online 2003; 7:515–542.
32. Stillman RJ, Richter KS, Banks NK, et al. Elective single embryo transfer: a 6-year progressive implementation of 784 single blastocyst transfers and the influence of payment method on patient choice. Fertil Steril 2009; 92:1895–906.
33. Practice Committee of Society for Assisted Reproductive Technology; Practice Committee of American Society for Reproductive Medicine. Elective single-embryo transfer. Fertil Steril 2012; 97:835–842.
34. Roberge S, Giguère Y, Villa P, at al. Early administration of low-dose aspirin for the prevention of severe and mild pre-eclampsia: a systematic review and meta-analysis. Am J Perinatol 2012; 29:551–556.
35. National Institute for Clinical Excellence (NICE). Hypertension in pregnancy: the management of hypertensive disorders during pregnancy. NICE clinical guideline CG107. London: NICE, 2010.
36. Royal College of Obstetricians and Gynaecologists (RCOG). Reducing the risk of thrombosis and embolism during pregnancy and puerperium. Green-top Guideline No. 37a. London: RCOG, 2009.
37. Nicolaides KH. Screening for fetal aneuploidies at 11–13 weeks. Prenat Diagn 2011; 31:7–15.
38. National Institute for Clinical Excellence (NICE). Antenatal care: routine care for healthy pregnant women. NICE clinical guideline CG62. London: NICE, 2008.
39. Zollner U, Dietl J. Perinatal risks after IVF and ICSI. J Perinat Med 2013; 41:17–22.
40. Van Voorhis BJ, Williamson RA, Gerard JL, et al. Use of oocytes from anonymous, matched, fertile donors for prevention of heritable genetic diseases. J Med Genet 1992; 29:398–399.

Chapter 10

Human papillomavirus and cervical cytology

Mehrnoosh Aref-Adib, Theresa Freeman-Wang

CERVICAL CANCER

Worldwide, cervical cancer is the fourth most common cancer in women. It is the most common cancer in women aged 15–44 years, accounting for 9% of new diagnoses, over 500,000 cases and over 266,000 deaths per year [1]. Of these, 28 000 deaths occur in Continental Europe. In the UK, both the incidence and deaths from cervical cancer have reduced since the introduction of a systematic cervical screening programme in 1988 [2]. Screening for cervical cancer differs from other cancer screening because there is a well-defined pre-malignant stage of disease which can be easily treated.

Cytology

In the 1920s Aurel Babes, and Georgiou Papanicolaou described the use of exfoliative cytology to identify women with cervical cancer. The technique, commonly referred to as a conventional or Papanicolaou (Pap) smear, gained popularity in the 1940s [3]. It involved placing a sample of fluid from the posterior vaginal fornix on a slide, which was then fixed with a Papanicoloau stain. Ayres refined the technique with a spatula to take a scrape of cells in the cervix, increasing the yield of cervical cells, which are then reviewed by a cytologist. This remained the standard screening tool for over 50 years until the advent of liquid based cytology. Studies had been reported showing a wide range of sensitivities (44–86%) and specificities (62–98%) for the Pap smear [4]. False negative rates could be as high as 50% [5, 6].

Liquid based cytology

Liquid based cytology (LBC) was developed to produce a more representative sample of the specimen than a conventional smear, and to reduce contamination by blood cells, pus and mucus [7]. It has been shown that LBC reduces the inadequate rate from 9 to 1.6%, increasing the productivity of laboratories and reducing women's anxiety and their need to return for repeat cytology.

Mehrnoosh Aref-Adib MBBS MA MRCOG, Queens Hospital, Romford, UK.

Theresa Freeman-Wang MBChB MRCOG, The Whittington Hospital, London, UK. Email: theresa.freeman-wang@nhs.net (for correspondence)

The two most widely studied technologies for LBC preparation are SurePath (formally Autocyte), (TriPath Imaging Inc.) and ThinPrep (Cytyc UK) [7]. LBC involves taking a sample of cells from the transformation zone of the cervix in a similar way to conventional cytology. The material obtained on the broom collection device is dispersed in a preservative fluid to generate a suspension of cells. In the lab, the suspension is centrifuged and passed through a filter to create a slide with a monolayer preparation of well-preserved cellular morphology [8].

The original Papanicolaou classification of cytology findings has largely been superseded. Currently there are two main classifications of cervical cytology. The Bethesda classification (2001) is widely used in many countries. This incorporates both cytological and histological change. Until 2013, the British Society of Clinical Cytology (BSCC) had a different categorisation. The latest revision is now more similar to the Bethesda system (see Table 10.1: differences in terminology).

Cytological abnormalities are described as dyskaryosis. This is an abnormal chromatin pattern, with the grade of dyskaryosis defined by determining the ratio of nuclear diameter to cytoplasmic diameter. Current definitions are given below and **Table 10.1** provides a comparison between previously used and current terms.

Cervical intraepithelial neoplasia

Cervical intraepithelial neoplasia (CIN) refers to the histological diagnosis of a spectrum of changes in squamous epithelium known to be precursors of invasive squamous cell carcinoma. There are three grades currently in use that reflect a continuum of epithelial change. The current grading system allows correlation with the three previous cytological grades of dyskaryosis – mild, moderate and severe dyskaryosis suggesting CIN1, CIN2 and CIN3 respectively (**Figures 10.1, 10.2, 10.3**) [9].

CIN1 may be difficult to distinguish from reactive and other non-neoplastic histological changes. The diagnosis of CIN3 is more robust than that of CIN1or CIN2. In CIN3, there is a full thickness abnormality with a degree of nuclear pleomorphism that is more severe when compared to two lower grades. There are a larger number of mitoses at all levels and the changes are seen extending to surface. There is very little, if any, cytoplasmic maturation present.

Table 10.1 Previous and new cytological terminology [9A]	
Previous terminology (BSCC 1986)	**New terminology**
Borderline change	Borderline change in squamous cells Borderline change in endocervical cells
Mild dyskaryosis Borderline change with koilocytosis	Low-grade dyskaryosis
Moderate dyskaryosis	High-grade dyskaryosis (moderate)
Severe dyskaryosis	High-grade dyskaryosis (severe)
Severe dyskaryosis ?Invasive	High-grade dyskaryosis/?invasive squamous carcinoma
?Glandular neoplasia	?Glandular neoplasia of endocervical type ?Glandular neoplasia (non-cervical)

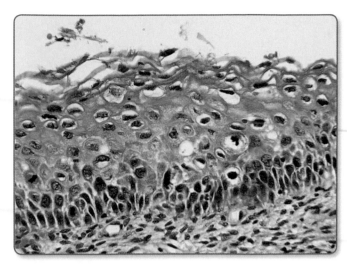

Figure 10.1 Image of CIN1. Basal 1/3 of epithelium occupied by abnormal cells (increased mitotic activity). By courtesy of the Whittington Hospital.

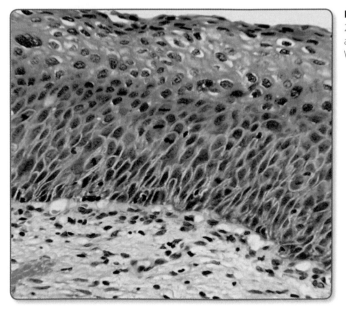

Figure 10.2 Image of CIN2. Basal 2/3 of the epithelium occupied by abnormal cells. By courtesy of the Whittington Hospital.

Squamous intraepithelial lesion (Bethesda 2001)

In the Bethesda classification abnormalities are described as either low-grade squamous intraepithelial lesion (LSIL) equivalent to CIN1 or high-grade squamous intraepithelial lesion (HSIL), equivalent to CIN2 and CIN3. In addition another term atypical squamous cells of unknown significance (ASCUS) is used. ASCUS has no direct equivalent in the UK classification, though borderline abnormalities are a close comparison. Both represent a class of smears with a low-risk of underlying CIN3 [10].

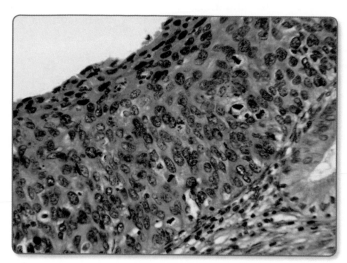

Figure 10.3 Image of CIN3. Full thickness of epithelium occupied by abnormal cells. By courtesy of the Whittington Hospital.

Cervical screening

Cervical screening was first introduced in British Columbia and Finland. It began in the UK in the 1960s. Implementation was opportunistic and did not significantly reduced cancer rates until 1988 when a systematic call and recall programme was developed [11]. It is now one of the most successful cancer prevention programmes.

Cervical screening saves approximately 4500 lives per year in England and in other countries with high population coverage from screening a 60–70% reduction in deaths has been seen [10, 12]. Mortality rates in 2008 (2.4 per 100,000 females) were nearly 70% lower than 30 years earlier (7.1 per 100,000 females in 1979) [2]. In 2011, there were 972 deaths from cervical cancer in the UK [13]. A total of 3.6 million women aged 25-64 years were tested in 2011–2012.

Primary screening

Coverage, which refers to the proportion of eligible women being screened in the previous 5 years, has remained fairly consistent in the UK over the last 20 years. There has been a gradual decline from 82% in the 1990s to 79% in the last 5 years [14].

In England, the first invitation occurs at 25 years of age. In other parts of the UK cervical screening begins at the age of 20 years. The age range was changed in England in 2003 because of concerns over treatment in young women with low grade or small volume premalignant lesions that would resolve spontaneously and because of fears related to subsequent pregnancy morbidity. Between the ages of 25-49 years subsequent invitations are distributed every 3 years. From 50-64 years, women are invited every 5 years. Women over 65 years are only invited if they have not been screened in the past or they have had recent abnormal cytology results tests. Women aged 65years or over whose last three consecutive adequate tests have been reported as negative are removed from the screening programme.

Secondary screening: colposcopy

Colposcopy, first described in 1925 by Hans Hinselmann, is the examination of the cervix with a lighted, low-powered microscope. Although colposcopy may be part of an annual general gynaecology assessment as in much of Continental Europe, it is predominantly a secondary screening tool used to determine appropriate management for women referred with an abnormal cytology result. A biopsy may be taken from the cervix for diagnosis and/ or the cervix may be treated. Alternatively, women may remain under surveillance and have repeated testing every 6–12 months. In the UK, approximately 150 000 referrals to colposcopy are made annually [15].

Human papillomavirus

In 1983 zur Hausen first isolated human papillomavirus (HPV) (type 16) from cervical carcinoma, which led to the identification of HPV as a potential causative organism for the development of cervical cancer [16]. It is predominantly sexually transmitted and a reflection of sexual activity, with a lifetime risk of up to 80% [16]. The prevalence of HPV declines with age (**Figure 10.4**) [7]. The infection is often an asymptomatic and transient event persisting in 10–15% of women [18]. Over 120 types of HPV have since been identified [19]. HPV types 16 and 18 are together responsible for 70–80% of cervical cancers and 50% of all premalignant change [17]. They also account for 40–50% of vulval and oropharyngeal cancers and 70–80% of anal cancer [20, 21]. More recently an expert panel have classified HPV types into five categories (**Table 10.2**) [22A].

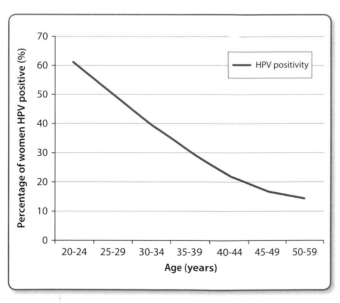

Figure 10.4 Declining prevalence of HPV positivity with increasing age [22B].

Table 10.2 Categorisation of HPV subtypes and pathogenesis		
Group	**Definition**	**HPV types**
Group 1	Carcinogenic to humans	16, 18, 31, 33, 35, 39, 45, 51, 52, 56, 58, 59
Group 2A	Probably carcinogenic to humans	68
Group 2B	Possibly carcinogenic to humans	53, 64, 65, 66, 67, 69, 70, 73, 82
Group 3	Not classifiable	6, 11
Group 4	Probably not carcinogenic	

Four stages of disease development have been described: HPV acquisition, HPV persistence, progression of persisting infection to precancer, and invasion (**Figure 10.5**) [23]. Natural history studies indicate that persistent infection is associated with a high relative risk of developing high-grade CIN [10]. The prevalence of infection in a 'normal' population will vary with age, being highest in younger women and decreasing up to age 45 years [7].

Factors known to affect the risk of HPV positivity are shown in **Table 10.3**. The postulated mechanisms by which current oral contraceptive use influences infection include the enhancing effect of oestrogens on cervical ectopy, thereby permitting potential carcinogens (including HPV) easier access to the transformation zone, and increased cell proliferation and transcription of HPV induced by direct hormonal effects on cervical cells [2,25].

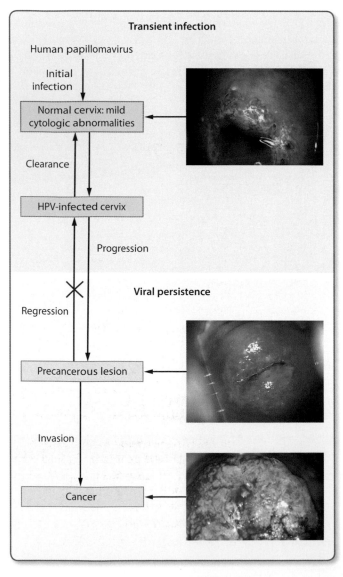

Figure 10.5 A simplified model of the natural history from HPV infection to the development of cervical cancer. Adapted from Wright T, Schiffman M. N Engl J Med 2003; 348:489-490. Photos courtesy of Whittington Hospital Colonoscopy Department.

Table 10.3 Aetiological factors associated with human papillomavirus (HPV) [24, 25]
Reduced HPV risk
Increasing age
Obtaining tertiary education
White ethnicity
Married/co-habiting status
Pregnancy resulting in childbirth (particularly if first pregnancy over 20 years)
Increased HPV risk
Lower age
Lower educational level
Non-white ethnicity, e.g. black-African, Indian, Pakistani
Single or divorced/separated/widowed
Current and previous oral contraceptive (OC) use (combined or progesterone-only)
Current use of other hormonal contraception (e.g. implants, injections, intrauterine system)
Current smoking status

Compared with never smokers, current smokers (but not ex-smokers) were at a modest increased risk, unrelated to smoking pack-years. Barrier contraception and physical activity were also unrelated to risk.

Human papillomavirus and men

Men are less likely to have persistent HPV and unlike in women, no association has been found with age. Circumcision, the use of condoms and reduced number of lifetime female sexual partners are thought to reduce the transmission of HPV to males [26,27]. Bosch reported that the presence of HPV in the husbands' penis conveyed a five-fold risk of cervical cancer to their wives [28].

Methods of human papillomavirus testing

The first clinically applied HPV detection methods in the 1980s included in situ hybridisation [29]. HPV has a stable double-stranded DNA genome that can be accessed easily from exfoliated cells [30]. Currently five techniques for detecting HPV are approved in the US for clinical use, including four DNA-based assays: digene Hybrid Capture 2 (HC2) (Qiagen NV, Venlo, Netherlands), Cervista HPV HR (Hologic Inc., Bedford, MA, USA), Cervista HPV 16/18 test (Hologic Inc., Bedford, MA, USA), Cobas 4800 HPV (Roche Molecular Diagnostics, Pleasanton, CA, USA); and one RNA assay: APTIMA HPV assay (formerly GenProbe Inc., San Diego, CA, USA).

Qiagen hybrid capture II is the gold standard HPV test and was the first reliable, quality standardised HPV DNA test. It works by hybridisation in solution of one strand of template DNA to complementary RNA probes of 13 different HPV types, and these types are responsible for the vast majority of cervical cancers [31]. In 2003, FDA approval was extended to the use of HC 2 alongside routine Pap testing for women over the age of 30 years [32]. There is a simpler version care HPV (Qiagen NV, Venlo, Netherlands), available for use in low resource settings.

The emergence of nucleic acid amplification techniques (NATs) has allowed for the development of alternative HPV detection assays beyond hybrid capture II.

Cervista is a signal amplification method that uses invader technology for the qualitative detection of 14 high-risk HPV type (Day). Using a Cleavase enzyme; 14 HR-HPVs can be detected.

Cobas 4800 HPV (Roche) detect HPV 16 and 18 individually and other HR-HPVs in aggregate and is suitable for cervical screening with risk stratification beyond presence/absence of HPV.

Aptima HPV (GenProbe now Hologic) detects 14 HR-HPV types by detecting mRNA. There is evidence of increased specificity, thus it may be particularly useful for HPV triage.

Roles of human papillomavirus testing

In clinical practice there are three roles for HPV DNA testing:
1. Primary screening for cervical neoplasia
2. In triage of minimally abnormal and inconclusive smears
3. As a 'test of cure' post treatment

Human papillomavirus as a primary screening test for cervical cancer

In 2006 an overview of the European and North American studies on primary cervical cancer screening reviewed over 60,000 women and demonstrated a sensitivity of 96.1% and specificity of 90.7% for HPV testing versus cytology which had a sensitivity of 53% and specificity of 96.3% [7]. A recent meta-analysis demonstrated that primary screening with HPV testing can allow for an increase in the interval between screening episodes of up to 6 years, which could offset the increased costs of new technology with less frequent screening [33]. The high positive rates for HPV testing in young un-immunised women limit the clinical effectiveness of primary HPV screening in the population under the age of 30 years [34]. However, the sentinel sites project of primary HPV screening is including women from the age 25 years to mirror the current English cervical screening programme.

Its potential value in a low resource setting was demonstrated by a study from rural India, which showed that a single round of HR-HPV testing by HC II was associated with a significant decline in the rate of advanced cervical cancers and associated deaths, compared with the unscreened control group [35]. A possible algorithm for the use of HPV testing as the sole primary screening modality is shown in **Figure 10.6**.

Human papillomavirus triage

HR-HPV prevalence in women with borderline smears varies within the studies from 31% to 72% [18, 36]. HPV testing of women with low-grade abnormal smears can separate those HPV negative women who are unlikely to have high-grade CIN from those who are HPV positive and therefore at higher risk.

Human papillomavirus studies

Although many studies have been undertaken the following four studies have provided the most robust evidence for the role of HPV in screening and triage. Following these studies HPV triage has been introduced in England (**Figure 10.7**).

ASCUS/LSIL triage study

ASCUS/LSIL triage study (ALTS) was a multicentre, randomised clinical trial designed to evaluate three alternative methods of management of ASCUS or LSIL, namely, immediate colposcopy, cytologic follow-up, and triage by HPV.

HPV-DNA testing (HC II) showed the highest sensitivity and identified 96.3% (95% CI 91.6–98.8) of women with CIN3+, which was at least as sensitive as an immediate

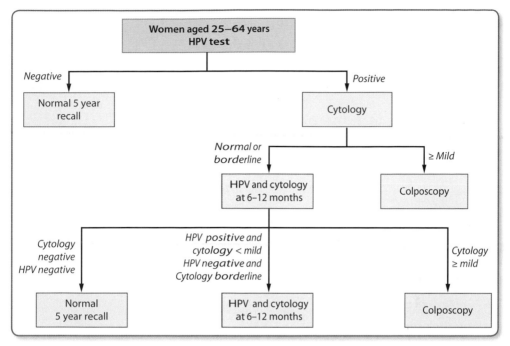

Figure 10.6 Primary HPV screening potential. A possible algorithm for the use of HPV testing as the sole primary screening modality for women ages 25–64 years, followed by Pap triage of HPV positive women. By courtesy of Professor Jack Cuzick.

colposcopy [37]. High sensitivity, combined with a reasonable specificity for triage, has made HPV-DNA testing the recommended option for the management of ASCUS cytology.

As 83% (82.9%) of patients with LSIL were positive for HPV, it was not considered useful for triage of this group. By contrast, in England, triage of this group has proved cost effective as 17% of women can be returned to normal recall rather than be referred for colposcopy [38].

The ALTS study also looked at variation in the interpretation of cytology samples. Substantial differences were found among expert pathologists in interpreting both thin-layer Pap tests and biopsies. Regarding the accuracy of colposcopy directed biopsy, this study found increased sensitivity when more than one biopsy was taken.

Trial of management of borderline and other low grade abnormal smears study [39–41][1]

The aims of this 7-year multicentre trial were:
1. To assess whether conservative management or immediate colposcopy was more effective in women with low-grade smear abnormalities.
2. To determine whether women should have immediate treatment with large loop excision of the transformation zone (LLETZ) or a colposcopy and directed biopsy with recall for treatment if the punch biopsy showed high grade disease.
3. To determine whether HPV testing added to the effectiveness of the current management of low grade smear abnormalities.

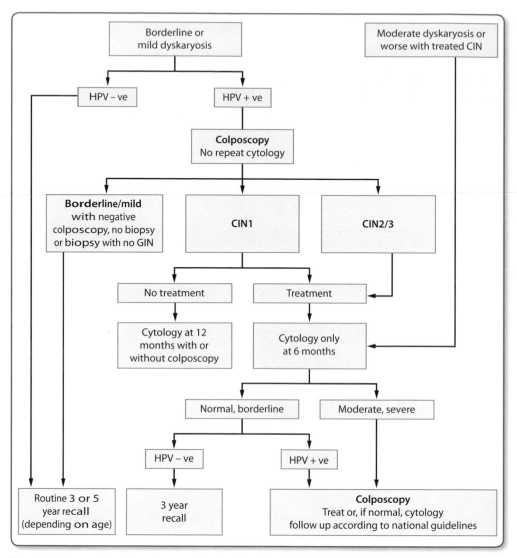

Figure 10.7 Protocol for HPV triage, currently in use in England. By courtesy of NHS Cancer Screening Programmes, part of the Health and Wellbeing Directorate of Public Health, England.

The study population comprised 10 000 women between the ages of 20 and 59 years with an index borderline test followed by another test, 6 months later, which showed either borderline or mild dyskaryosis. Cytological screening was performed every 6 months in primary care (n = 2223) or patients were referred for colposcopy and related interventions (n = 2216). All women were followed for 3 years. Among women randomised to immediate colposcopy, 79% (74.9–82.5%) of cases of CIN2 or worse were diagnosed. Of women randomised to cytological surveillance a similar number 77% (72.1–81.2%) of cases were detected by surveillance cytology and related interventions.

The trial recommended a policy of surveillance rather than triage for two reasons; the first was that some CIN2 will regress with time and the second was that they identified a high proportion of HPV-negative CIN2. The authors demonstrated the ability to return to recall not only 50% of those referred to colposcopy but also the 35% of women who were HPV-negative based on HPV triage [39–41].

A randomised trial of HPV testing in primary cervical screening (ARTISTIC trial) [18, 42]

This trial investigated HPV as a primary screening tool. In addition it sought to review cost and psychological implications of adding HPV testing to cytology.

Twenty-five thousand women aged 20–64 years attended general practices for routine cervical screening and who consented to having an HPV test. There were two interventions: Cervical cytology plus HPV (revealed) versus cytology alone (HPV testing performed, but result concealed) and these were evaluated over two screening rounds, 3 years apart.

Round 1 detected prevalent disease and round 2 a combination of incidence and undetected disease from round 1. HPV testing was performed on the LBC sample obtained at screening.

In round 1, women were randomised in a ratio of 3:1 to either have the HPV test result revealed (and acted upon if persistently positive in cytology-negative cases) or concealed. There was no difference in CIN3+ between the arms when rounds 1 and 2 were combined. The HPV-positive rate was 31.1% for borderline cytology and 69.9% for mild dyskaryosis. The study found that the prevalence of HR-HPV types was age-dependent, and that overall prevalence of HPV16/18 increased with the severity of dyskaryosis.

The accuracy of LBC was not improved from with the addition of HPV testing. However, an initial negative HPV test provided the same degree of 'protection' (negative predictive value) over two screening rounds as negative cytology for one screening round. This would allow the screening interval to be increased to 5–6 years or longer in women over 30 years of age. No significant adverse psychosocial effects of HPV testing were detected. The authors concluded that it would not be cost-effective to screen with cytology and HPV combined, but HPV testing, as either triage or initial test triaged by cytology, would be cheaper than cytology without HPV testing.

Sentinel site project [38]

In 2001, the HPV/LBC pilot studies reported on the feasibility of introducing HPV triage in the English screening programme [7]. Three sites converted to using LBC and HPV triage with the HC II assay for women with borderline cytology or mild dyskaryosis. Initially all HPV-positive women were referred to colposcopy, whereas HPV negative women were re-tested at 6 months and referred to colposcopy if they were HPV positive or had mild dyskaryosis. The results suggested that although HPV triage decreased the number of repeat cytology tests and reduced the time taken to return women to routine recall, it resulted in a large increase in referrals to colposcopy. It was however feasible, acceptable to women and cost-effective [7, 43].

As a result, HPV implementation was piloted in 6 sentinel sites throughout England to determine the effect of national rollout [38]. All women aged 25–64 years with routine cytology reported as borderline or mild dyskaryosis were eligible for inclusion in the study. Women who tested negative for HPV were returned to routine recall at 3 years or 5 years depending on their age and women positive for HPV were referred for colposcopy without repeat cytology.

Of the 10051 women eligible for inclusion into the study, 6507 had borderline cytology and 3544 had mild dyskaryosis. HPV positive rates were 53.7% in women with borderline cytology and 83.9% for women with mild dyskaryosis. Of those HPV positive women who attended colposcopy 54.6% had no CIN, 16.3% had CIN2 or worse and 6.1% had CIN3 or worse. There were three cases of cervical cancer, all in women aged 25–34 years.

Human papillomavirus as a test of cure post treatment

Women who have had treatment for CIN or early stromal cancer remain at risk of recurrence [44]. In a meta-analysis of 28 studies, the extent of treatment failures was estimated to range from 7.1–11.3% [34]. Given the high sensitivity and negative predictive value of HPV testing, its incorporation into post treatment algorithms can significantly reduce the number of patients requiring follow-up [30].

Arbyn et al analysed the studies in which the HC2 assay was used for monitoring purposes in patients after treatment of CIN. Treatment failure expressed in terms of residual or recurrent CIN occurred in 10.2% (95% CI 6.7–13.8) of treated cases. Despite data heterogeneity, the pooled HR-HPV-DNA results after treatment predicted residual/recurrent CIN with a significantly higher sensitivity than conventional cytology-based follow-up. Overall, the combination of HR-HPV-DNA testing and cytology demonstrated a 96% sensitivity (95% CI 89–99), 81% specificity (95% CI 77–84), 46% PPV (95% CI 38–54) and 99% NPV (95% CI 98–100) [45].

The sentinel sites study also looked at 'test of cure' post treatment. At 6 months after treatment if cytology was reported as normal, borderline or mildly dyskaryotic and the HPV was negative, they were referred back to 3- yearly recall in the community. If cytology was reported as normal, borderline or mildly dyskaryotic and HPV was positive, they were referred to colposcopy. 25.7% of women treated (107/416) 'failed' test of cure; 15.6% due to an abnormal cytology and 10.1% due to a positive HPV test. The rate of failure decreased with increasing severity of CIN grade treated. Of the 107 women who failed test of cure, 41 attended a subsequent colposcopy; 65.9% of women were negative for CIN, however 12.2% tested positive for CIN2 or worse. Overall the positive predictive value of HPV infection in cytologically negative women for detecting residual CIN3 or worse was 0.4%, for detection of CIN2 or worse was 2.9% [38].

Other uses of human papillomavirus testing

Human papillomavirus in the resolution of uncertainties

HR-HPV testing may be of use in the following clinical scenarios [46]:
1. In women under long-term surveillance for low grade CIN
2. Cervical stenosis
3. Colposcopy is unsatisfactory
4. Those with a persistent mismatch between high-grade cytology and low-grade histology.

Human papillomavirus and glandular abnormalities

The incidence of invasive and preinvasive glandular lesions of the uterine cervix has been increasing. Cervical cytology was designed to detect squamous rather than glandular abnormalities. Despite this, glandular abnormalities are an important category as it may be a sign of noncervical malignant change including endometrial or ovarian cancer.

For women with a glandular abnormality, conisation with close surveillance, including repeat cytology, colposcopy, punch biopsy and endocervical curettage is frequently recommended.

Unfortunately, the conservative management of glandular lesions has a substantial false negative rate [48]. Following treatment, there is a 15% rate of recurrence compared with 5% for squamous abnormalities. For this reason, hysterectomy is usually considered once a woman's family is complete.

Costa and colleagues found that the combination of HC2 and cytology reached 90% sensitivity in detecting persistent lesions at the first follow-up visit and 100% sensitivity at the second among women treated conservatively for adenocarcinoma in situ or adenocarcinoma [48]. This may prove a more robust method of follow up for these lesions.

Developments in human papillomavirus testing

Self-sampling human papillomavirus testing

Self-taken samples usually comprise swabs placed in a suitable viral transport medium, but dry brushes, urine and Guthrie-type filter paper have also been investigated [49]. HPV self-tests are commercially available and may eventually help screen coverage. In 2007 Szarewski et al evaluated the self-test and found it to be highly acceptable. In 921 women, the sensitivity of the self-test for high grade HPV was 81% and found to be higher than that of the cytology self-test (48%) [50].

The psychosexual morbidity associated with positive HPV test results must be considered. Women who discover they have an untreatable sexually transmitted infection that increases their risk of cancer may suffer from low self-esteem and marital problems (even though such a positive test may never result in significant pathology) [10]. Thus, the availability of the test outside a screening programme is a cause for concern, as there is no current mechanism for those with a positive result to be assessed in a quality assured system.

Genotyping

As HPV positivity is so common, there is an increasing need to look for other prognostic markers to assist management and identify those most at risk of high grade pre-malignancy. The American Society for Colposcopy and Cervical Cytology (ASCCP) screening guidelines include genotyping in the management algorithm for cytology negative and HR-HPV-DNA positive patients [51]. Women with evidence of HPV 16 and/or 18 are recommended for immediate colposcopy, whilst those who have one of the other HR-HPV types are kept under annual cytological and HPV surveillance.

Emerging markers for human papillomavirus

One of the most established biomarkers for HPV is $p16^{INK}$ – a cyclin-dependent kinase inhibitor that regulates the cell cycle. HPV protein upregulates $p16^{INK}$ and $p16^{INK}$ levels are known to increase with increasing severity of disease. Tsoumpou et al showed that 2%, 38%, 68% and 82% of normal, CIN1, CIN2 and CIN3 were positive for $p16^{INK}$. In addition, cases of CIN1 that were $p16^{INK}$ negative were found less likely to progress [52].

Other cellular markers indicative of HPV-associated neoplasia include Topoisomerase IIa (TOP2A), minichromosone maintenance proteins (MCMs), MYBL2 and Survivin. Furthermore, there is evidence that the methylation of CADM1 (host) and L1 and L2 genes (virus), which is associated with a worse prognosis, may represent a potential marker [53].

Human papillomavirus vaccination

It is anticipated that vaccination will have a considerable impact on the prevalence of cervical cancer. There is already evidence of this from Australia, which was the first country to offer widespread HPV vaccination. There are two licensed virus-like particle vaccines: Gardasil (Sanofi Pasteur MSD Ltd, Maidenhead, Berks, UK), a quadrivalent vaccine covering HPV 16/18/6/11 and Cervarix (GlaxoSmithKline, Uxbridge, Middlesex, UK), covering HPV 16/18. Both vaccines are given as three doses over a 6-month period, with safety and efficacy demonstrated by a number of phase III trials [54]. Completion of all three vaccinations is necessary to effectively reduce the risk of cervical cancer [55]. It is predicted that vaccination will reduce the incidence of, and morbidity associated with premalignant cervical disease. Vaccination is also predicted to affect other cancers associated with HPV [17].

The Papilloma Trial against Cancer In young Adults (PATRICIA) was an international, Phase III, double-blinded, multicentre RCT [56]. The study involved the vaccination of HPV negative women with either cervarix in the treatment group, or hepatitis A vaccine as a control. The study found the vaccine was 94.2% effective in preventing CIN2.

Despite the advantages of the vaccination program, the cost of treatment and the acceptability of vaccinating young girls and ineffectiveness against established HR-HPV are seen as possible disadvantages.

Therapeutic human papillomavirus vaccination

Significant progress is being made in preclinical models of a vaccine to treat existing HPV related cervical lesions, which have resulted in several early phase clinical trials. The aim of therapeutic vaccination is to eliminate pre-existing lesions by generating cellular immunity against HPV-infected cells.

Key points for clinical practice

- HPV is necessary but not sufficient to cause cervical cancer.
- 80–90% of the population will have an HPV infection at some point in their reproductive lives. For most people HPV is a transient infection that will clear over an average of 3 years (median 18 months to 2 years).
- There is increasing evidence that high risk HPV are associated with other lower genital tract cancers and oropharyngeal tumours.
- Vaccination may help to reduce the burden of HPV 16 and 18 but it will remain important for women to have cervical screening for the foreseeable future.
- HPV 16 and 18 account for 70–80% of cervical cancer, 40–50% of vulval cancers, 40–50% of oropharyngeal cancers and 70–80% of anal cancer.
- HPV testing has been shown to be of value in the triage of low grade smear abnormalities. It has been adopted as part of NHSCSP since 2012.
- Scotland, Wales and Northern Ireland have different programmes. Trials for primary HPV screening have commenced in England and are likely to begin in Scotland.

REFERENCES

1. World Health Organization International Agency on Research for Cancer. GLOBOCAN 2012: estimated Cancer Incidence, Mortality and Prevalence Worldwide in 2012. http://globocan.iarc.fr/Pages/fact_sheets_cancer.aspx. Last accessed 31/10/13.
2. Cervical cancer incidence statistics. London: Cancer Research UK. Available at www.cancerresearchuk.org/cancer-info/cancerstats/types/cervix/incidence/#trends. Last accessed November 2013.
3. Papanicolaou GN, Traut HF. The diagnostic value of vaginal smears in carcinoma of the uterus. Am J Obstet Gynecol 1941; 42:193–206.
4. International Agency for Research on Cancer (IARC), World Health Organization. Chapter 2, Screening tests. In: IARC handbooks of cancer prevention, volume 10: cervix cancer screening. Lyon: IARC Press, 2005.
5. Guidos BJ, Selvaggi SM. Use of the Thin Prep Pap Test in clinical practice. Diagn Cytopathol 1999; 20:70–3.
6. Papillo JL, Zarka MA, St John TL. Evaluation of the Thin Prep Test in clinical practice; a seven-month, 16, 314-case experience in northern Vermont. Acta Cytol 1998; 42:203–208.
7. Moss SM, Gray A, Marteau T, et al. Evaluation of HPV/LBC cervical screening pilot studies. Report to the Department of Health (Revised October 2004). Available from www.cancerscreening.nhs.uk/cervical/evaluation-hpv-2006feb.pdf, last accessed February 2013.
8. Abulafia O, Pezzullo.JC, Sherer DM. Performance of ThinPrep liquid-based cervical cytology in comparison with conventionally prepared Papanicolaou smears: a quantitative survey. Gynecol Oncol 2003; 90:137–144.
9. Shingleton HM, Richart RM, Wiener J, et al. Human cervical intraepithelial neoplasia: fine structure of dysplasia and carcinoma in situ. Cancer Res 1968; 28:695–706.
9A. John HF, Patnick, J (eds.) for NHS Cervical Screening Programme. Achievable standards, benchmarks for reporting, and criteria for evaluating cervical cytopathology, Third edition including revised performance indicators. Sheffield; NHS Cancer Screening Programmes, 2013.
10. Kitchener H. The value of human papillomavirus testing. Obstet Gynaecol 2003; 5:10–13.
11. Albrow R, Kitchener H, Gupta N, et al. Cervical screening in England: the past, present, and future. Cancer Cytopathol 2012; 120:87–96.
12. Peto J, Gilham C, Fletcher O, et al. The cervical cancer epidemic that screening has prevented in the UK. Lancet 2004; 364:249–256.
13. Cervical cancer mortality statistics: http://www.cancerresearchuk.org/cancer-info/cancerstats/types/cervix/mortality/. Last accessed November 2013.
14. Patrick J (ed.). NHS Cervical Screening Programme 2012. Annual Review. Sheffield: NHS Cervical Screening Programmes, 2012.
15. Health and Social Care Information Centre, Screening and Immunisations Team. Cervical Screening Programme, England, 2011–2012. Leeds: Health and Social Care Information Centre, 2012.
16. Dürst M, Gissmann L, Ikenberg H, et al. A papillomavirus DNA from a cervical carcinoma and its prevalence in cancer biopsy samples from different geographic regions. Proc Natl Acad Sci USA 1983; 80:3812–3815.
17. Fiander A. Prophylactic human papilloma virus vaccination update. Obstet Gynaecol 2009; 11:133–135.
18. Kitchener HC, Almonte M, Wheeler P, et al. HPV testing in routine cervical screening: cross-sectional data from the ARTISTIC trial. Br J Cancer 2006; 95:56–61.
19. Bernard HU, Burk RD, Chen Z, et al. Classification of papillomaviruses (PVs) based on 189 PV types and proposal of taxonomic amendments. Virology 2010; 401:70–79.
20. Brabin L, Fairbrother E, Mandal D, et al. Biological and hormonal markers of chlamydia, human papillomavirus, and bacterial vaginosis among adolescents attending genitourinary medicine clinics. Sex Transm Infect 2005; 81:128–132.
21. Moscicki AB, Shiboski S, Broering J, et al. The natural history of human papillomavirus infection as measured by repeated DNA testing in adolescent and young women. J Pediatr 1998; 132:277–284.
22A. Bouvard V, Baan R, Straif K, et al. A review of humancarcinogens – Part B: biological agents. Lancet Oncol 2009; 10:321–322.
22B. Cotton SC, Sharp L, Seth R, et al. Lifestyle and socio-demographic factors associated with high-risk HPV infection in UK women. Br J Cancer 2007; 97:133–139.
23. Cuzick, Clavel C, Petry KU, et al. Overview of the European and North American studieson HPV testing in primary cervical cancer screening. Int J Cancer 2006; 119:1095–1101.

24. Green J, Berrington de Gonzalez A, Smith JS, et al.Human papillomavirus infection and use of oral contraceptives. Br J Cancer 2003; 88:1713–1720.

25. de Villiers EM. Relationship between steroid hormone contraceptives and HPV, cervical intraepithelial neoplasia and cervical carcinoma. Int J Cancer 2003; 103:705–708.

26. Nielson CM, Schiaffino MK, Dunne EF, et al. Associations between male anogenital human papillomavirus infection and circumcision by anatomic site sampled and lifetime number of female sex partners. 2009; 199: 7–13.

27. Nielson CM, Harris RB, Dunne EF, et al. Risk factors for anogenital human papillomavirus infection in men. J Infect Dis 2007; 196:1137–1145.

28. Bosch FX, Castellsagué X, Muñoz N, et al. Male Sexual Behavior and Human Papillomavirus DNA: Key Risk Factors for Cervical Cancer in Spain, J Natl Cancer Inst 1996; 88:1060–1067.

29. Cubie HA, Norval M. Detection of human papillomaviruses in paraffin wax sections with biotinylated synthetic oligonucleotide probes and immunogold staining. J Clin Pathol 1989; 42:988–991.

30. Cubie HA, Cuschieri K. Understanding HPV tests and their appropriate applications. Cytopathology 2013; 24:289–308.

31. Origoni M, Cristoforoni P, Costa S, et al. HPV-DNA testing for cervical cancer precursors: from evidence to clinical practice ecancer 2012; 6:258.

32. FDA approved device: http://www.fda.gov/medicaldevices/productsandmedicalprocedures/deviceapprovalsandclearances/recently-approveddevices/ucm082556.htm.

33. Arbyn M, Martin-Hirsch P, Buntinx F, et al. Triage of women with equivocal or low-grade cervical cytology results: a meta-analysis of the HPV test positivity rate. J Cell Mol Med 2009; 13:648–659.

34. Arbyn M, Ronco G, Anttila A, et al. Evidence regarding human papillomavirus testing in secondary prevention of cervical cancer. Vaccine 2012; 30:F88–99.

35. Sankaranarayanan R, Nene BM, Shastri SS, et al. HPV screening for cervical cancer in rural India. N Engl J Med 2009; 360:1385–1394.

36. Cuschieri KS, Cubie HA, Whitley MW, et al. Multiple high risk HPV infections are common in cervical neoplasia and young women in a cervical screening population. J Clin Pathol 2004; 57:68–72.

37. Solomon D, Schiffman M, Tarone R. Comparison of three management strategies for patients with atypical squamous cells of undetermined significance: baseline results from a randomized trial. J Natl Cancer Inst 2001; 93; 293–299.

38. Kelly RS, Patnick J, Kitchener HC, et al. HPV testing as a triage for borderline or mild dyskaryosis on cervical cytology: results from the Sentinel Sites study. Br J Cancer 2011; 105:983–988.

39. TOMBOLA Group. Biopsy and selective recall compared with immediate large loop excision in management of women with low grade cervical cytology referred for colposcopy: mulitcentre randomised controlled trial. BMJ 2009; 339:b2549.

40. TOMBOLA Group. Cytological surveillance compared with immediate referral for colposcopy in management of women with low grade cervical abnormalities: multicentre randomised controlled trial. BMJ 2009b; 339:b2546.

41. TOMBOLA Group. Options for managing low grade cervical abnormalities detected at screening: cost effectiveness study. BMJ 2009c; 339: b2549.

42. Kitchener HC, Almonte M, Gilham C, et al. ARTISTIC: a randomised trial of human papillomavirus (HPV) testing in primary cervical screening. Health Technol Assess 2009; 13:1–150.

43. Legood R, Gray A, Wolstenholme J, et al. Lifetime effects, costs, and cost effectiveness of testing for human papillomavirus to manage low grade cytological abnormalities: results of the NHS pilot studies. BMJ 2006; 332:79–85.

44. Costa S, De Nuzzo M, Infante FE, et al. Disease persistence in patients with cervical intraepithelial neoplasia undergoing electrosurgical conization. Gynecol Oncol 2002; 85:119–124.

45. Arbyn M, Paraskevaidis E, Martin-Hirsch P, et al. Clinical utility of HPV-DNA detection: triage of minor cervical lesions, follow-up of women treated for high-grade CIN: an update of pooled evidence. Gynecol Oncol 2005; 99:S7–11.

46. Smith JHF, Patrick J (eds). Achievable standards, benchmarks for reporting, and criteria for evaluating cervical cytopathology. NHSCSP Publications 20, 3rd edn. January 2013. Sheffield: NHS Cervical Screening Programmes, 2013.

48. Costa S, Negri G, Sideri M, et al. Human papillomavirus (HPV) test and PAP smear as predictors of outcome in conservatively treated adenocarcinoma in situ (AIS) of the uterine cervix. Gynecol Oncol 2007; 106:170–176.

49. Virtanen A, Nieminen P, Luostarinen T, et al. Self-sample HPV tests as an intervention for non-attendees of cervical cancer screening in Finland: a randomized trial. Cancer Epidemiol Biomarkers Prev 2011; 9:1960–1969.

50. Szarewski A, Cadman L, Mallett S, et al. Human papillomavirus testing by self-sampling: assessment of accuracy in an unsupervised clinical setting. J Med Screen 2007; 14:34–42.

51. Saslow D, Solomon D, Lawson HW, et al. American Cancer Society, American Society for Colposcopy and Cervical Pathology, and American Society for Clinical Pathology Screening Guidelines for the Prevention and Early Detection of Cervical Cancer. Journal of Lower Genital Tract Disease 2012; 16: 175-204.

52. Zhang Q, Kuhn L, Denny LA, et al. Impact of utilizing p16INK4A immunohistochemistry on estimated performance of three cervical cancer screening tests. Int J Cancer 2007; 120:351–356.

53. Wentzensen N, Bergeron C, Cas F, et al. Triage of women with ASCUS and LSIL cytology: use of qualitative assessment of p16INK4a positive cells to identify patients with high-grade cervical intraepithelial neoplasia. Cancer 2007; 111:58–66.

54. FUTURE II Study Group. Quadrivalent vaccine against human papillomavirus to prevent high-grade cervical lesions. N Engl J Med 2007; 356:1915–1927.

55. Garland SM, Hernandez-Avila M, Wheeler CM, et al. Quadrivalent vaccine against human papillomavirus to prevent anogenital diseases. N Engl J Med 2007; 356:1928–1943.

56. Paavonen J, Naud P, Salmerón J, et al. HPV PATRICIA Study Group. Efficacy of human papillomavirus (HPV)-16/18 AS04-adjuvanted vaccines against cervical infection and precancer caused by oncogenic HPV types (PATRICIA): final analysis of a double-blind, randomised study in young women. Lancet 2009; 25; 374:301–314.

Chapter 11

Prostaglandins and parturition

Natalie C McKirdy, Hassendrini N Peiris, Greg E Rice, Murray D Mitchell

BIOSYNTHESIS AND REGULATION

The term eicosanoid applies to all metabolites of arachidonic acid; these molecules have similar chemical structures with subtle differences, depending upon their parent molecule – two-arachidonoyl glycerol, arachidonic acid, or anandamide (**Figure 11.1**).

Arachidonic acid-derived eicosanoids

Phospholipids from cell membranes are cleaved by either the direct action of phospholipase A_2 or indirectly by the action of phospholipase C and diacyl- and mono-acylglycerol lipase (DAGL and MAGL, respectively), resulting in the release of arachidonic acid and lysophospholipid. Arachidonic acid is converted to the intermediate PGH_2 by one of two isoforms of cyclo-oxygenase (COX), also known as prostaglandin H synthase (PGHS); the constitutive COX-1 (PGHS-1), or inducible COX-2 (PGHS-2) (**Figure 11.1**). This is considered to be rate-limiting step in the eicosanoid biosynthesis cascade. PGH_2 is further modified by terminal synthases to create the prostaglandins (PGD_2, PGE_2, $PGF_{2\alpha}$ and PGI_2), or thromboxane A_2 (TXA_2) (**Figure 11.1**) [1].

The endocannabinoid converter, fatty acid amide hydrolase

Anandamide is the precursor of prostamides (PMs) (**Figure 11.1**). The enzyme fatty acid amide hydrolase (FAAH) readily converts anandamide to arachidonic acid, providing the substrate for labour-promoting prostaglandin (PG) production. As one would expect, anandamide concentrations are elevated in the uterus and placenta of FAAH knockout mice when compared to the wild-type control [2]. The absence of FAAH restricts anandamide metabolism to its own pathway (**Figure 11.1**), driving prostamide (PM) production rather than PG production.

Natalie C McKirdy BSc, University of Queensland Centre for Clinical Research, Royal Brisbane & Women's Hospital Campus, Queensland, Australia. Email: natalie.mckirdy@uq.edu.au (for correspondence)

Hassendrini N Peiris MSc, University of Queensland Centre for Clinical Research, Royal Brisbane & Women's Hospital Campus, Queensland, Australia.

Gregg E Rice PhD Grad Dip MGT MAH BSc(Hons), University of Queensland Centre for Clinical Research, Royal Brisbane & Women's Hospital Campus, Queensland, Australia.

Murray D Mitchell MD D Phil D.Sc FRSNZ, University of Queensland Centre for Clinical Research, Royal Brisbane & Women's Hospital Campus, Queensland, Australia.

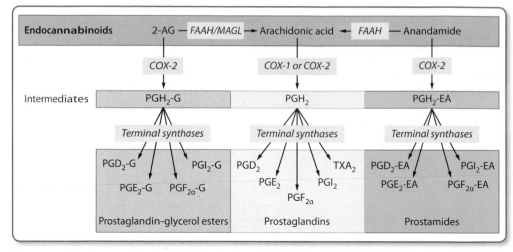

Figure 11.1 The eicosanoid biosynthesis pathway, demonstrating relationships between eicosanoid species and the enzymes involved. 2-AG; 2-arachidonoylglycerol, FAAH; fatty acid amide hydrolase; MAGL, monoacylglycerol lipase; COX, cyclo-oxygenase (isoforms 1 and 2). As an example of metabolite nomenclature, PGH_2; prostaglandin H_2, or its similar derivatives from 2-AG (PGH_2-G, prostaglandin H_2 glycerol ester), and anandamide (PGH_2-EA, prostaglandin H_2 ethanolamide). Enzyme names italicised and shaded grey.

The rate of biosynthesis, and by extension, the concentration, varies depending upon the eicosanoid, tissue/location, and gestational time-point. Concentrations of eicosanoids, their precursors, metabolites, and regulating factors have been investigated to varying degrees, in an effort to determine normal concentrations for each stage of gestation. Challis et al. proposed that maturation of the fetus influences initiation of labour through activation of the fetal hypothalamic-pituitary-adrenal axis [3]. Increasing cortisol production from the fetal adrenal gland is common in the animal model, yet a synchronous increase in adrenal oestrogen precursor nearing term was restricted to primates. Despite mechanisms differing between sheep and primate models, the outcome is identical: placental and intrauterine tissues increase production of oestrogen approaching the end of gestation. Challis et al. propose that fetal cortisol acts on the placenta to increase prostaglandin H synthase (PGHS) expression and activity, thereby increasing PG concentration within the fetal membranes [3]. In addition, fetally-derived cortisol may retard the metabolism of PGs within this region, allowing concentrations to rise within proximal tissues to maximally assert the PG autocrine/paracrine function. Elevated production of corticotropin-releasing hormone (CRH) may also feed into this system [3].

In most animals, a functional withdrawal of progesterone towards term signals imminent labour onset, however, such withdrawal does not occur in humans. Some hypothesise that the high progesterone level that coincides with labour is necessary for the opposing activity between upper and lower regions of the uterus: the fundus undergoing contractions while the cervix and nearby myometrial tissue relaxes to facilitate the expulsion of the fetus [3].

There is no one cause for preterm labour; the maturation of the hypothalamic-pituitary-adrenal axis may be asynchronous to the rest of the fetus, causing the onset of labour and delivery prior to, or after, term; another proposed activator is an ascending intrauterine infection whereby the associated leukocyte infiltration into uterine tissues brings about cytokine and other pro-inflammatory mediator production in the immediate area [4]. The resultant inflammatory response, driven in part by the eicosanoids produced, is thought to be instrumental to labour initiated in this manner [4]. Researchers are working to profile the physiological, and in some cases pathological, causes of mistimed labour with a view to earlier diagnoses allowing closer management of pregnancies at risk of preterm delivery.

Endocannabinoids and their metabolites – the prostaglandin glycerol esters, prostaglandins, and prostamides – deliver their cellular function via cell surface receptors (Figure 11.2); although they are specific, receptor subtypes occur for some PGs, e.g. PGE_2 may bind to EP_1-EP_4. The ratios of expression of the receptors vary between tissues, which enable the range of tissue-specific PG responses [4].

Prostaglandins (PGs) and other eicosanoids act in opposing ways to co-ordinate balance, or homeostasis. Whilst some PGs promote vascular dilation, others promote constriction; some promote inflammation and yet others, its inhibition; even sleep versus wakefulness [4]. Studies have found that the balance is disrupted in pathological processes such as pre-eclampsia and cardiovascular disease and that the discordant concentrations can be exacerbated or mitigated through exposure to specific cytokines or inhibitors [4].

Evidence is mounting that pro-inflammatory mediators, such as interleukin-1β and others present in an infection-induced preterm labour, instructs transcription of the gene required for prostacyclin synthase (PGES). Many biological systems observe the pro-inflammatory milieu preceding and promoting simultaneous up-regulation of

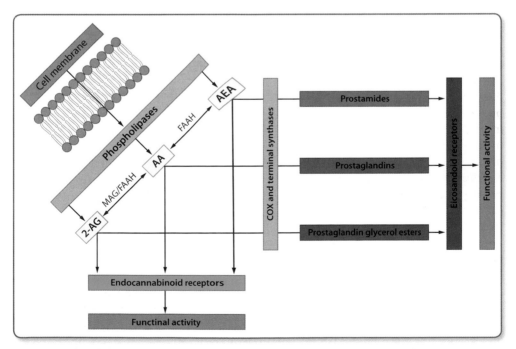

Figure 11.2 Phospholipases act on cell phospholipid bilayers to liberate the endocannabinoids 2-arachidonoylglycerol (2-AG); arachidonic acid (AA); and anandamide (AEA) – the precursors of prostamides, prostaglandins and prostaglandin-glycerol esters. An endocannabinoid can be modified into its sister molecule by the action of monoacylglycerol lipase (MAGL) or fatty acid amide hydrolase (FAAH). While the endocannabinoids exert a biological function themselves, they can be further modified by cyclo-oxygenases (COX-1 or -2) and terminal synthases to produce highly specialised functional activities.

membrane-bound PGES (mPGES) coupled to an increase in COX-2, producing PGE_2 [4]. The COX-2:mPGES coupling has been implied in the increase in PGE_2 immediately preceding ovulation, and cytosolic PGES (cPGES) is expressed in murine uterine tissues prior to implantation, suggestive of a role in implantation success and, due to the balanced nature of prostanoid actions, may also be important for decidualisation when fertilisation does not occur [4]. Until recently, little was known about the specific effects of each PGES pertaining to gestation and labour, other than these basic interrelationships.

Prostacyclin synthase and cyclo-oxygenase-2

As gestation progresses and labour advances, COX-2 expression and activity in fetal/maternal membranes increases. By extension, mPGES is boosted and PG biosynthesis increases, with the major site of PGE_2 production being the amnion [3]. The highest frequency of immunoreactive mPGES was in the amnion epithelium and chorion laeve trophoblasts, whilst the decidua showed low or no detectable immunoreaction [5]. Similar examination of the placenta found that mPGES enzyme occurred at low levels in the syncytiotrophoblast and cells proximal to blood vessels, but was mPGES protein increased in the chorion but decreased in placenta during labour [5]. This led the investigators to suggest that mPGES may be differentially regulated during labour. Similar to mPGES, cPGES was found in the amnion epithelium, but also in the fibroblasts and macrophages in the chorion trophoblast layer [6]. When examined by Western blot, no difference was found in protein level expression between the two synthases with respect to term or preterm labour. This suggests that PGE_2 biosynthesis is rate-limited at a point higher up in the metabolic pathway; Helliwell et al. proposed that this may occur at the COX-2 or cPLA-2 level [7]. There was, however, a change in distribution pattern of both synthases from a cytosolic dispersion at preterm, to clustered at term associated with lipid droplets, the contents of which are yet to be determined [6]. PGE_2 has a widely accepted role in stimulation of myometrial contractions, but due to its many subtypes of receptor and differential expression of the same, PGE_2 could well have further actions in pregnancy and parturition presently currently unknown, such as the recently discovered PGE_2 stimulation of matrix metalloproteinase 9 in fetal membranes in vitro [8].

Prostaglandin F$_2$ alpha synthase (PGFS)

Prostaglandin $F_{2\alpha}$ ($PGF_{2\alpha}$) increases at parturition and is known to affect myometrial contraction and cervical relaxation, but little is known of the regulation and expression of its synthase, PGFS, during pregnancy [7]. When ovine distribution of $PGF_{2\alpha}$ mRNA was investigated and compared to COX-2 by Wu et al, it was found in all tissues examined (myometrium, endometrium, maternal and fetal placenta in induced preterm labour and spontaneous term labour). Interestingly, both betamethasone-induced preterm labour and spontaneous labour at term showed an increase in COX-2 but not PGFS mRNA [9]. This indicates that the rate-limiting step in increasing $PGF_{2\alpha}$ is not transcription.

Prostacyclin synthase (PGIS) and thromboxane synthase (TXAS)

Prostacyclin or prostaglandin I_2 (PGI_2) has powerful smooth muscle relaxant effects, yet it has long been identified as a major stimulator of uterine contractions, and is the main eicosanoid found in myometrial tissue of pregnant animals, including humans [3]. These seemingly contradictory effects may be explained by the differential expression of subtypes of PGI receptors between regions of tissues. Its terminal synthase, PGIS, has been observed in pregnant and non-pregnant ovine tissues and found to be differentially regulated during labour. Inflammatory cytokines, in particular tumour necrosis factor-α (TNFα), interleukin-1α (IL-1α), IL-1β, and IL-6, are known to increase PGI production by inducing expression of PGIS mRNA and protein [7].

The ratio of PGI to TXA is thought to be important for homeostasis *in vivo* as they act in opposition to each other. Upon immunohistochemical staining, PGI was seen localised in the endothelial cells within the placental villi, whereas TXA was found in the trophoblasts, which implicates their roles in the fetal side and maternal side of placental circulation, respectively [10].

Maternal plasma concentrations of PGI increase during parturition, yet PGIS concentration in myometrial myocytes and vascular smooth muscle cells and endothelial cells from the lower uterine segment was found to be inversely proportional to advancing gestational age. Instead, cyclic mechanical stretch of the myometrial tissues may induce PGIS expression, triggering release of PGI, as was found to be the case *in vitro* [11].

Prostaglandin-D synthase (PGDS)

Prostaglandin D_2 (PGD$_2$) is produced in large amounts by the human placenta when subjected to superfusion conditions in vitro, and smaller amounts were liberated by gestational membranes [7]. Macrophages, which are known to invade the myometrium in readiness for onset of labour at term, are another important source of PGD$_2$. In addition to these mechanisms, laminar shear stress stimulates release of PGD$_2$ and upregulates expression of the secreted, lipocalin-type PGDS in human umbilical vein endothelial cells.

BIOLOGICAL FUNCTIONALITY

Eicosanoids (including prostaglandins) and endocannabinoids affect their biological activity by binding to G-protein-coupled receptors (GPCRs). Depending upon whether the GPCR contains a G_i or G_s protein, cyclic adenosine monophosphate (cAMP) production is inhibited or stimulated, respectively.

Prostaglandin E_2 (PGE$_2$), e.g. may bind to any of four GPCRs, (EP1, EP2, EP3 or EP4) working to increase cAMP if bound to EP2 or EP4, but decrease cAMP if bound to EP3. These modulations in cAMP concentrations eventually up-regulate COX-2 gene expression and feedback into the regulatory system [12].

Due to their contractile action on myometrium and cervical ripening activity, prostaglandins are an ideal candidate for gynaecological applications. Procedures such as cervical preparation for nulliparous post-menopausal hysteroscopy [13], medical termination of pregnancy [14], and management of missed miscarriage [15] have all benefited from advances in the understanding of prostaglandin interactions with the tissues and signalling systems of the female reproductive system. Each of the aforementioned applications in the reproductive system relies on the ripening and contractive effects that prostaglandins have on the cervical and myometrium, respectively.

MECHANISMS OF ACTION THROUGHOUT PREGNANCY

Early pregnancy miscarriage

Endocannabinoids and their receptors play a large role in co-ordinating development and implantation of embryos, and are similarly involved in onset of labour and miscarriage.

Low or absent fatty acid amide hydrolase

Expression of FAAH mRNA and activity of the protein itself in peripheral lymphocytes was significantly reduced in women who went on to spontaneously miscarry or experience an IVF pregnancy which failed in the first trimester, compared to levels in tissues collected from gestational age-matched pregnancies which underwent voluntary termination and pregnancies which continued as normal, to term [16, 17]. Immunohistochemically, FAAH could not be detected by staining trophoblast cells from first trimester miscarriages, but was seen in trophoblasts from voluntary termination placentae [18]. However, another study found no difference in FAAH expression in trophoblast cells between normal pregnancy and recurrent miscarriage, but did find FAAH to be elevated in the decidual stromal cells of women who repeatedly miscarried compared to normal pregnancy placental tissues [19]. In addition, mice lacking the ability to express FAAH (FAAH knockout murine model) experienced preterm labour [20]. In this way, low or no FAAH activity has been linked to early uterine stimulation, loss of pregnancy, and labour onset.

We propose, in the case of low or no FAAH, that anandamide is unable to be readily converted by FAAH activity to the PG precursor, arachidonic acid. Anandamide levels accumulate, and drive the production of PMs, changing the prostaglandin:prostamide (PG:PM) ratio and stimulating uterine contractions. In support of this, PMs $F_{2\alpha}$, E_2, and D_2 concentrations were found to be at least three-fold greater in FAAH knockout mice after administering anandamide, than the wild-type controls [21]. One can conclude from these findings that interactions of FAAH and anandamide are important for normal progression of pregnancy, and that decreased or absent FAAH activity leads to increased PM concentrations with detrimental effects on the pregnancy. For these reasons, anandamide and FAAH may be candidates for biomarker analysis of placental dysfunction and adverse pregnancy outcomes.

Labour onset and progression

The exact pathways critical to the onset of labour are yet to be established; this is due, in no small part, to the fact that many of the cell types found in fetal membranes are able to produce the factors suggested to be involved in parturition, and is compounded by the heterogeneity of those tissues denying researchers the ability to attribute production to discrete areas or layers of tissue.

Endocannabinoids in labour onset via PG production

Endocannabinoids promote labour through production of PGs. PGs are lipid molecules that play a critical role in the mechanisms of miscarriage and parturition at both term and preterm [3]. Recently, the first data were published in evidence of endocannabinoids and synthetic cannabinoids stimulating fetal membrane production of PGE_2 in a CB1-dependent manner [22]. Similar findings were generated by another group using rat uterus exposed to anandamide to increase PGE_2 and $PGF_{2\alpha}$, this time in a CB2 receptor-dependent manner [23]. PGE and PGF are associated with the regulation of myometrial contractions, cervical ripening, and membrane rupture. PG-related compounds, such as prostacyclins and thromboxanes, contribute to these changes, but have also been found to coordinate in the vasculopathy of pre-eclampsia [3, 24].

Olson and Amman outlined five distinct, sequential physiological events of parturition [26]; Rupture of the fetal membranes, dilation of the cervix, contraction of the myometrium, separation of the placenta, and uterine involution – all involve PGs, but the most extensively studied area of PG involvement is in myometrial contractility. The return to quiescence via involution, however, is thought to be mainly orchestrated by oxytocin. Terzidou outlined the involvement of eicosanoids such as prostaglandin or prostacyclin (PGI_2), along with other 'pro-labour' factors including relaxin, nitric oxide, oxytocin receptors, CRH, and parathyroid hormone-related peptide (PTHrP), in the progressing phases of parturition [25].

During uterine quiescence, PGI_2, relaxin, nitric oxide and act through a variety of mechanisms, to increase the concentration of cAMP or cyclic guanosine monophosphate (cGMP) within the cells, preventing release of intracellular calcium, denying activation of myosin light chain kinase, and hence, inhibiting myometrial contractions [26].

Activation of uterine function occurs with the involvement of prostaglandins. CRH and oestrogen rise during this phase, which, with the possible inclusion of mechanical stretch, triggers the expression of genes requisite for contractions, namely prostaglandins, connexin 43, and oxytocin receptors. CRH receptors, expressed on by both myometrium and fetal membranes, are bound to cAMP-second messenger G proteins, causing upregulation of COX-2 expression, thus positively feeding back into the pathway to produce more prostaglandins.

The same urotonins – prostaglandin, oxytocin, and CRH – are responsible for the stimulation phase, whereby the intrauterine biochemistry closely resembles an inflammatory response. Cytokine IL-8 is known to attract neutrophils into the cervix, and also induce PGE_2 production. At this stage, prostaglandins are responsible for ripening the cervix, relaxing the lower portion of the uterus, and stimulating contractions in the upper segment (fundus).

POTENTIAL DIAGNOSTIC ABILITY OF EICOSANOIDS

Cross-reactivity in previous detection methods

The generation of antibodies for immunological methods of detection (enzyme linked and radiolabelled immunoassays) is not a precise science. In order to illicit an immune response and raise antisera, the small lipid structures (eicosanoids) are conjugated to a larger molecule (bovine serum albumin, BSA) at their point of difference – the polar head group (Figure 11.3c). Antibodies can be generated against any part of the target molecule, but when conjugated thus, antibodies detect areas nearer the conjugation site poorly, and favour molecules similar to the antigen (target molecule). Hence, if two or more molecules share a similar structure, there is a high-risk of cross-reactivity. For instance, prostamide E_2 (PME_2) has a larger functional group at its carboxyl terminus than PGE_2, so not only will an antibody raised against PGE_2 recognise and bind PME_2 due it its similarity in structure, it will bind more avidly to it because, having a larger functional group, it more closely resembles the conjugated antigen against which it was raised [26].

With the homology displayed by the eicosanoid family due to their common precursor, there is a very small region of distinction between each compound, and hence, and a large potential for cross-reactivity among antibodies generated against these molecules. This has caused misleading data and incorrect conclusions to be drawn in the past, as was evidenced by examining commercial antisera raised against BSA-conjugated PGs which demonstrated major cross-reactivity with prostamides (Figure 11.3a and b) [26]. The study also found evidence that anandamide metabolism by cell line and primary amnion tissue

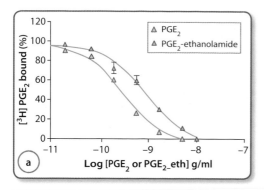

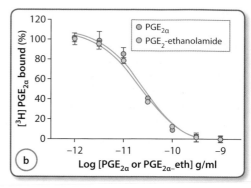

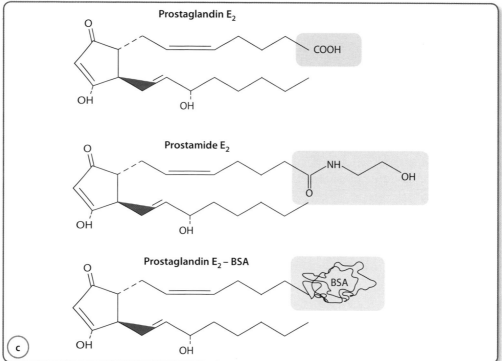

Figure 11.3a–c Cross-reactivity of prostamides with prostaglandins. Standardised prostaglandin radioimmunoassays were used to determine the ability of prostamides to displace tritiated prostaglandin from the antibody compared with the parent compound. (a) Displacement of [3H] prostaglandin E_2 (PGE_2) from in-house-generated antibody by PGE_2 (closed triangles) or PGE_2-ethanolamide (PGE_2-eth; open triangles). (b) Displacement of [3H] prostaglandin $F_{2\alpha}$ ($PGF_{2\alpha}$) from anti-$PGF_{2\alpha}$ antibody by $PGF_{2\alpha}$ (open circles) or $PGF_{2\alpha}$-ethanolamide ($PGF_{2\alpha}$-ethanolamide; closed circles). Error bars represent standard error of the mean (With permission from Glass et al., 2005). (c) The similarity between structures of prostamide E_2 (PME_2), prostaglandin E_2 (PGE_2), and the antigenic prostaglandin E_2–BSA (bovine serum albumin) conjugate, highlighting the size and location of functional groups. Note that prostamide E_2 is more similar to the commonly used antigen (PGE_2-BSA) than PGE_2 itself, due to the larger moiety at the carboxyl end. Modified from McKirdy et al, 2013.

explants, in the presence of cytokine stimulation, produced a predominately PM output rather than PGs [26]. This was only discovered, however, after separation by thin layer chromatography, because the metabolites were first measured by radioimmunoassay and were detected as PGs. Hence, it is possible that in inflammatory reactions, the substrate is converted to PM rather than PG.

With respect to PTL research, accurate detection of eicosanoids is paramount; the major identifiable cause of PTL is intrauterine infection [27], which may trigger increased production of PMs which, with previous popularity of antibody-base detection methods, may have largely been misidentified as PGs. PM precursor, anandamide, has been shown to be released in cases of haemorrhagic shock [28] and exposure of macrophages and human peripheral lymphocytes to lipopolysaccharide [29]. Similarly, $PGHS_2$ is increased in response to inflammatory mediators including IL-1α and lipopolysaccharide [30]. The concurrent increase in both anandamide and $PGHS_2$ could direct and increase in PME_2.

These findings imply that reliance on antibody-based methods for detection and quantification of PGs are lacking in specificity, and could be masking a diagnostically useful change in the PG:PM ratio (Figure 11.4). Instead, physical detection methods such as chromatography and mass spectrometry would be better employed in the role of detection and quantification of eicosanoids, on the basis of their specificity and sensitivity. Only then will we be able to accurately define the temporal relationships at play within the complex system, as the variability in previous measurements may have been entirely due to changes in the PG:PM ratio. Now, with the ability to physically detect these compounds, we may be able to separate normal fluctuations from pathological concentrations of these bioactive lipids, potentially harnessing them as a diagnostic for PLT risk.

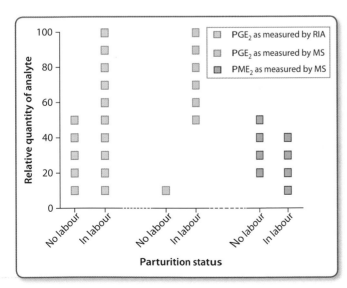

Figure 11.4 Demonstration of the diagnostic benefit of the higher specificity mass spectrometry (MS) method of prostaglandin and prostamide detection and quantitation, versus antibody-based methods, e.g., radioimmunolabelled assay (RIA). Determining concentration based on the interaction of the molecular structure with a calibrated, reproducible, consistent ionisation beam, rather than interaction with a biologically derived, and hence, inherently inconsistent antibody, enables reliable separation of signal into individual eicosanoid species, e.g. prostaglandin E$_2$ (PGE$_2$) and prostamide E$_2$ (PME$_2$). This enables researchers to attribute the change in concentration between non Labour and Labour states to changes in specific eicosanoids. Note: Graph depicts a hypothetical data set. With permission from Chan et al, 2013.

CONCLUSION

Compiling an analyte profile for informing preterm labour

From analysis of the literature, we can draw together a profile of changes in expression and concentration of certain analytes which may be strongly indicative of risk of preterm labour. A profile is necessary because of the complexity of the labour induction pathway, e.g. alone, high plasma anandamide levels are not enough to characterise risk of PTL; depending on the concentrations and activities of other analytes, increased anandamide may have a stimulatory or inhibitory effect on labour. Such are the paradoxical clinical indications of elevated anandamide in pregnancy.

High plasma anandamide concentration and reduced PGHS activity

Reduced (or absent) FAAH activity leads to reduced conversion of anandamide to arachidonic acid, which limits substrate availability for conversion to PGs. As PGs have a strong stimulatory effect on myometrial contractions, one may conclude that low FAAH activity would cause low PG concentrations, decreasing the risk of spontaneous labour but, if PGHS is not available for metabolism to PMs, high plasma anandamide concentrations can increase CB receptor expression in placental tissues **(Figure 11.5)**. CB1 was found to be elevated in spontaneous miscarriage, and has been linked to uterine PGE_2 production; in

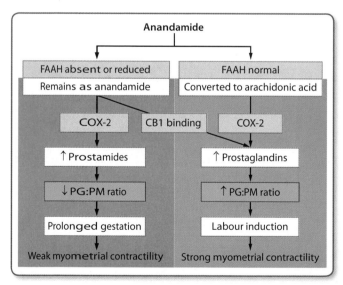

Figure 11.5 A new model for the spontaneous onset of preterm labour. The model implies that anandamide metabolism effects the prostaglandin:prostamide (PG:PM) ratio. The presence or absence of fatty acid amide hydrolase (FAAH) and cyclo-oxygenase-2 (COX-2) are variable, which may lead to three possible outcomes: If FAAH is absent or reduced, anandamide is unable to be converted to arachidonic acid which increases the anandamide concentration. The elevated anandamide may (i) be metabolised by COX-2, which would increase prostamide production and therefore delay labour induction and prolong gestation, or (ii) bind the CB1 receptor, which our laboratory has shown to stimulate prostaglandin production, leading to an increased PG:PM ratio and labour induction. Lastly, (iii) in the case of normal or increased FAAH, anandamide may be converted to arachidonic acid, increasing the availability of prostaglandin substrate, and in doing so, increasing the PG:PM ratio and causing labour induction. By this logic, the PG:PM ratio may be useful as a biological marker for risk of initiation of uterine contractions. With permission from from Chan et al, 2013 [31].

this way, elevated plasma anandamide concentration may induce labour via PGE_2 [16–18]. Conversely, lacking CB1 receptors or being treated with CB1 receptor agonists caused mice to display preterm onset of labour compared to normal and CB2 receptor knockout mice.

High plasma anandamide concentration in the presence of active PGHS

If the increased anandamide concentration occurs in the presence of PGHS, it can be metabolised to PMs, driving the PG:PM ratio down, and will have only a weak stimulatory effect on uterine contractions and may even prolong gestation (**Figure 11.5**). Clearly, regulation of the CB mechanisms in normal pregnancy is extremely tight, as variation from the physiological norm in either direction, results in pathological activity.

How we propose to use eicosanoids to determine risk/ presence of preterm labour

Due to cross-reactivity of PG and PM species giving rise to erroneous data interpretation from antibody-based detection methods, it is possible that a potentially clinically useful role for PGs as diagnostic and predictive factors for PTL has been missed in past investigations. Advances in mass spectrometry, however, mean that this issue can now be addressed.

Increased intrauterine PG production is considered a critical step in the onset of labour; This, coupled with the revelation of PMs formerly masked presence, the subsequent investigation of PM biological activity within reproductive tissues, and the definition of factors related to dynamics of eicosanoid production have led to the hypothesis that a panel of preterm labour biomarkers may allow earlier detection and more definitive risk analysis of PTL. Overall, the current literature informs potential biomarkers for risk of PTL as being FAAH, COX, PG:PM, CRH, relaxin, PTHrP, oxytocin receptors, anandamide and CB receptors. It has also demonstrated why measurement by methods that do not rely upon antibodies (i.e. mass spectrometry) is optimal for obtaining data and conclusions which accurately describe and reflect the true biological processes at play.

Future studies would ideally define, for each potential biomarker, the magnitude at which divergence from the normal gestational range indicates significant risk of PTL, the positive predictive value of each biomarker, and the most efficient combination. Detection of pathological changes at the earliest possible gestational age would confer maximum benefit, informing clinicians of the need for a higher level of patient management. Ultimately, this would enable a prophylactic tocolytic to be administered prior to onset of PTL to improve neonatal morbidity and mortality rates. As such, further research may identify a tocolytic effective in humans with fewer adverse effects than those currently available [25].

Key points for clinical practice

- Previous measurements of how prostaglandin concentration changes at the time of labour and delivery are methodologically confounded.

REFERENCES

1. Woodward DF, Liang Y, Krauss AH. Prostamides (prostaglandin-ethanolamides) and their pharmacology. Br J Pharmacol 2008; 153:410–419.
2. Sun X, Xie H, Yang J, et al. Endocannabinoid signaling directs differentiation of trophoblast cell lineages and placentation. Proc Natl Acad Sci USA 2010; 107:16887–16892.
3. Challis JRG, Matthews SG, Gibb W, et al. Endocrine and paracrine regulation of birth at term and preterm. Endoc Rev 2000; 21:514–550.
4. Hansen WR, Keelan JA, Skinner SJ, et al. Key enzymes of prostaglandin biosynthesis and metabolism. Coordinate regulation of expression by cytokines in gestational tissues: a review. Prostaglandins Other Lipid Mediat 1999; 57:243–257.
5. Alfaidy N, Sun M, Challis JR, et al. Expression of membrane prostaglandin E synthase in human placenta and fetal membranes and effect of labor. Endocrine 2003; 20:219–225.
6. Meadows JW, Eis AL, Brockman DE, et al. Expression and localization of prostaglandin E synthase isoforms in human fetal membranes in term and preterm labor. J Clin Endocrinol Metab 2003; 88:433–439.
7. Helliwell RJ, Adams LF, Mitchell MD. Prostaglandin synthases: recent developments and a novel hypothesis. Prostaglandins Leukot Essent Fatty Acids 2004; 70:101–113.
8. McLaren J, Taylor DJ, Bell SC. Prostaglandin E(2)-dependent production of latent matrix metalloproteinase-9 in cultures of human fetal membranes. Mol Hum Reprod 2000; 6:1033–1040.
9. Wu WX, Ma XH, Yoshizato T, et al. Increase in prostaglandin H synthase 2, but not prostaglandin F2alpha synthase mRNA in intrauterine tissues during betamethasone-induced premature labor and spontaneous term labor in sheep. J Soc Gynecol Investig 2001; 8:69–76.
10. Shellhaas CS, Coffman T, Dargie PJ, et al. Intravillous eicosanoid compartmentalization and regulation of placental blood flow. J Soc Gynecol Investig 1997; 4:58–63.
11. Korita D, Sagawa N, Itoh H, et al. Cyclic mechanical stretch augments prostacyclin production in cultured human uterine myometrial cells from pregnant women: possible involvement of up-regulation of prostacyclin synthase expression. J Clin Endocrinol Metab 2002; 87:5209–5219.
12. Klein T, Shephard P, Kleinert H, et al. Regulation of cyclo-oxygenase-2 expression by cyclic AMP. Biochim Biophys Acta 2007; 1773:1605–1618.
13. Kant A, Divyakumar, Priyambada U. A randomized trial of vaginal misoprostol for cervical priming before hysteroscopy in postmenopausal women. J Midlife Health 2011; 2:25–27.
14. Kulier R, Kapp N, Gülmezoglu AM. Medical methods for first trimester abortion. Cochrane Database Syst Rev 2011; 9:CD002855.
15. Neilson JP, Gyte GM, Hickey M, et al. Medical treatments for incomplete miscarriage. Cochrane Database of Systematic Reviews, 2013; 28;3:CD007223.
16. Maccarone M, Bisogno T, Valensise H, et al. Low fatty acid amide hydrolase and high anandamide levels are associated with failure to achieve an ongoing pregnancy after IVF and embryo transfer. Mol Hum Reprod 2002; 8:188–195.
17. Maccarone M, Valensise H, Bari M, et al. Relation between decreased anandamide hydrolase concentrations in human lymphocytes and miscarriage. Lancet 2000; 355:1326–1329.
18. Trabucco E, Acone G, Marenna A, et al. Endocannabinoid system in first trimester placenta: low FAAH and high CB1 expression characterize spontaneous miscarriage. Placenta 2009; 30:516–522.
19. Chamley LW, Bhalla A, Stone PR, et al. Nuclear localisation of the endocannabinoid metabolizing enzyme fatty acid amide hydrolase (FAAH) in invasive trophoblasts and an association with recurrent miscarriage. Placenta 2008; 29:970–975.
20. Wang H, Xie H, Guo Y, et al. Fatty acid amide hydrolase deficiency limits early pregnancy events. J Clin Invest 2006; 116:2122–2131.
21. Weber A, Ni J, Ling KH, et al. Formation of prostamides from anandamide in FAAH knockout mice analyzed by HPLC with tandem mass spectrometry. J Lipid Res 2004; 45:757–763.
22. Mitchell MD, Sato TA, Wang A, et al. Cannabinoids stimulate prostaglandin production by human gestational tissues through a tissue-and CB1-receptor-specific mechanism. Am J Physiol Endocrinol Metab 2008; 294:E352–E356.
23. Sordelli MS, Beltrame JS, Cella M, et al. Cyclo-oxygenase-2 prostaglandins mediate anandamide-inhibitory action on nitric oxide synthase activity in the receptive rat uterus. Eur J Pharmacol 2012; 685:174–179.
24. Walsh SW, Wang Y. Maternal perfusion with low-dose aspirin preferentially inhibits placental thromboxane while sparing prostacyclin. Hypertens Pregnancy 1998; 17:203–215.

25. Olson DM, Ammann C. Role of the prostaglandins in labour and prostaglandin receptor inhibitors in the prevention of preterm labour. Front Biosci 2007;12:1329–13243.
26. Glass M, Hong J, Sato TA, et al. Misidentification of prostamides as prostaglandins. J Lipid Res 2005; 46:1364–1368.
27. Romero R, Munoz H, Gomez R, et al. Does infection cause premature labor and delivery? Semin Reprod Med 1994; 12:227–239.
28. Wagner JA, Varga K, Ellis EF, et al. Activation of peripheral CB1 cannabinoid receptors in haemorrhagic shock. Nature 1997; 390:518–521.
29. Liu J, Batkai S, Pacher P, et al. Lipopolysaccharide induces anandamide synthesis in macrophages via CD14/MAPK/phosphoinositide 3-kinase/NF-κB independently of platelet-activating factor. J Biol Chem 2003; 278:45034–45039.
30. Lin CC, Sun CC, Luo SF, et al. Induction of cyclo-oxygenase-2 expression in human tracheal smooth muscle cells by interleukin-1beta: involvement of p42/p44 and p38 mitogen-activated protein kinases and nuclear factor-kappaB. J Biomed Sci 2004; 11:377–390.
31. Chan HW, McKirdy NC, Peiris H, et al. The role of endocannabinoids in pregnancy. Reproduction 2013; 146:R101-9.

Chapter 12

The use of adjuvant therapy in assisted reproductive technology

Ying C Cheong

INTRODUCTION

Unrealistic beliefs and expectations are somewhat reflected in the widespread use of many adjuvant and alternative treatments in the 21st century within the realms of assisted reproductive technology (ART).

Unfortunately for many, reproductive science is still in its infancy; for every couple that enjoys the success of assisted conception as a means of conception, many more face the distraught of failed treatments. In 2012, according to the European Society of Embryology and Reproduction, 1.5 million ART cycles were conducted globally and 1.1 million failed (76.7%). In 2010, in the United States, data from the centres for disease control indicated that 150,000 cycles were performed and 103,000 failed (68.6%). Such as many facets of medicine, where treatment success is limited and where world-leading scientists and medical specialists are still grasping with the lessons learnt from failures related to the medical science, many (patients and doctors) adopt the use of adjuvant and alternative treatments in the hope of bolstering the meager success of the therapy.

Many adjuvant and complementary treatments in ART are based on biological plausibility rather than evidence of efficacy, nevertheless there has been, in the recent decades, an increasingly avid use of adjuvant and complementary therapies in assisted conception. The purpose of this chapter is to provide a critically appraised evidence based overview of the currently used adjuvant and complementary treatment in assisted conception treatment.

HORMONES

Growth hormone

It is known that growth hormone (GH) regulates the effect of follicle-stimulating hormone (FSH) on granulosa cells, by increasing the synthesis of insulin-like growth factor-1, augments the effect of gonadotropin on granulosa and theca cells, and plays an essential

Ying C Cheong MB ChB BAO MA MD MRCOG, University of Southampton and Complete Fertility Centre Southampton, Princess Anne Hospital, Southampton, UK. Email: y.cheong@soton.ac.uk (for correspondence)

role in ovarian function, including follicular development, oestrogen synthesis and oocyte maturation[1]. Some studies have demonstrated that GH is associated with improvement in embryo quality, and high concentrations of GH in follicular fluid are related to good embryo morphology and increased rates of embryo implantation [2]. However, the data from randomised studies thus far has yielded conflicting results; some studies suggesting a potential benefit in the improvement in oocyte yield [3] and live birth rate [4] whilst others not [5, 6] . A meta-analysis of six relevant randomised controlled trials (RCTs) (n = 169) suggested that GH addition increased the probability of clinical pregnancy and live birth in poor responders undergoing ovarian stimulation with **gonadotropin-releasing hormone** (GnRH) analogues and gonadotrophins for **in vitro fertilisation** (IVF) although the reviewers cautioned the interpretation of the data due to the small sample size analysed [7]. Thus, routine use of GH on IVF patients cannot be recommended based on this data alone.

Androgens and androgen modulating agents

Androgens may play a role augmenting the response of poor responders to gonadotropin stimulation by increasing the number of primary, preantral and antral follicles independent of gonadotrophins [8], acting synergistically with FSH to increase follicular recruitment and granulosa cell proliferation [9]. Androgen-modulating agents such as letrozole and anastrozole are highly selective, non-steroidal aromatase inhbitors which blocks the conversion of androgen substrate to oestrogen in the granulosa cells and thereby increasing raised intraovarian androgens. A meta-analysis of 2481 cycles of IVF did not show any significant difference in the number of oocytes retrieved and on-going pregnancy/live-birth rates with androgen supplementation or modulation compared with the control groups [10] although a sensitivity analysis performed in this study highlighted that use of testosterone patches or DHEA has associated with an increased clinical pregnancy rate compared with controls (RR 2.86, 95% CI 1.73, 4.73). However, a more recent study based on 200 IVF cycles did not find any significant difference in the clinical pregnancy and miscarriage rates between women pre-treated with DHEA compared to those without DHEA pre-treatment (RR 1.87, 95% CI 0.96–3.64; and RR 0.59, 95% CI 0.21–1.65, respectively) [11]. Based on the results of the studies presented, routine use of androgens and androgen modulating agents cannot be recommended.

ANTICOAGULATION

Low-molecular-weight heparin (LMWH) is a commonly used form of thromboprophalaxis administered as a daily self-administered subcutaneous injection. LMWH does not require close monitoring due to its low side effects profile when compared with the traditionally used unfractionated heparin. Heparin is a structural analogue of heparan sulphate, one of the key components in implantation and early pregnancy events and is highly expressed throughout the reproductive tract. As heparin is highly anionic, it has high binding affinity, and can bind and modulate a wide range of molecular and cellular factors involved in implantation and trophoblastic differentiation and invasion. The use of heparin in women undergoing assisted reproductive treatment without thrombophilia is, however, still controversial. There has yet been no consensus as to the type of heparin, dose and duration of use if this treatment was to be used with ART patients. A recent Cochrane review [12]based on three studies (386 women) indicated that peri-implantation LMWH administration during assisted reproduction was associated with a significant improvement in live birth rate compared with placebo or no

LMWH [odds ratio (OR) 1.77, 95% confidence interval (CI) 1.07–2.90] side effects were poorly reported but included bruising and bleeding in the treated group. The authors emphasised the very low quality of the studies included, with high heterogeneity, and concluded that further studies were required to confirm this finding, and that routine use of heparin in ART patient is not justified outside the realms of research.

IMPROVING THE ENDOMETRIAL ENVIRONMENT

Endometrial biopsy

The relationship between endometrial injury and successful implantation was first observed in animal models and has subsequently been examined in clinical studies in different IVF populations. It is thought that this effect is related to the induction of local inflammation, which is conducive to implantation. Recent evidence suggests that local endometrial injury doubles the live birth rate of women undergoing IVF (13–15). A recent Cochrane review based on 591 women reported that endometrial injury in a previous cycle significantly increased the odds of live birth (OR 2.46, 95% CI 1.28–4.72). It did not recommend performing the endometrial injury during oocyte retrieval due to a significantly lower clinical pregnancy rate in one study (OR 0.30, 95% CI 0.14–0.63) [15]. The studies included however were clinically heterogeneous in terms of the number of biopsies performed per participant, the timing of the biopsies, the clinical characteristics of the participants included, and the type of biopsy catheter used. It seems that the procedure is best performed using an endometrial pipelle sampler transcervically and during the luteal phase in the prior cycle to the index IVF cycle. However, there is yet no consensus as to how extensive the endometrial biopsy should be, and whether the same applies to frozen embryo transfer cycles. Many IVF centres perform 'trial embryo transfers' on their patients prior to their IVF cycles, and in this context, given the relatively low side effects of endometrial injury pipelle biopsy, such a procedure could potentially be performed concurrently during the 'trial embryo transfer' in the luteal phase of the cycle before.

Vasodilators and muscle relaxants

Nonphysiological contractions of the myometrium have been observed both during and after embryo transfer. The effect may be secondary to the supraphysiological concentrations of steroid hormones that occur in an ovarian stimulation cycle, and also done to mechanical interruption of the uterine environment created by the process of embryo transfer itself. Vasodilators and uterine relaxing agents such as nitroglycerin/nitric oxide/sildenafil and β2-adrenergic antagonists (e.g. atosiban) have been studied in attempts to limit the possible adverse impact of uterine contractility. However, there is no evidence to support the routine use of these agents at and around the time of embryo transfer [16].

IMMUNOTHERAPY

Corticosteroids

Uterine receptivity may be modulated by locally acting growth factors and cytokines within the intrauterine environment [17, 18]. A defective integrity of this network of cytokines or an excess of NK cell activity has been implicated in implantation failure and recurrent miscarriage. The immunomodulation activity of corticosteroids is thought to improve the intrauterine environment by reducing the NK cell count and normalise the cytokine expression profile in the endometrium and by suppression of endometrial inflammation. However, the use of glucocorticoids have not been shown to improve pregnancy outcomes in women undergoing IVF/intracytoplasmic sperm injection (ICSI) although a subgroup analysis based on six studies and 650 women suggested that there may be borderline beneficial effect when corticosteroids were used in women undergoing IVF alone rather than IVF/ICSI (OR 1.50, 95% CI 1.05–2.13)[19, 20]. However, the studies included in the meta-analysis were heterogeneous, with variation in the type of corticosteroids used, the dosage, the timing, duration and mode of administration of the steroids. The adverse effects of steroids treatment were also poorly reported. Given the current evidence available and the potential side effects, the use of steroids during ART should be individualised.

Intravenous immunoglobulin and intralipid

The mode of action of the above products is far from being understood. Possible actions include alteration in NK cell activity and function as well as auto-antibody production. Intravenous immunoglobulin (IVIG) is a form of pooled blood product obtained from donor blood. The cost of this product varies from £1000–£1500 per infusion and the number of infusions per woman varies between 1–4 per ART cycle. It is therefore an expensive product, and carries risk of blood product related adverse reactions and transmission of viral/prion diseases. Intralipid, a 20% intravenous fat emulsion containing soybean oil, egg yolk, phospholipids, glycerine and water, normally used by patients requiring total parental nutrition costs approximately £200–£400 and has crept into the market as a 'safer' and 'cheaper' replacement of IVIG. Intralipid is normally given at a dose of 100 mL of 20% product diluted in 250 mL or 500 mL of normal saline infused over 1–2 hours. There is currently no evidence for the use of these products in ART and many authorities such as the British Fertility Society, NICE and the Department of Health, UK [16, 21, 22] do not recommend their use in ART patients.

TRADITIONAL CHINESE MEDICINE

Acupuncture and herbal medicine

Acupuncture is an integral part of traditional Chinese medicine (TCM) and has been used for at least 3000 years. In Europe, from consumer surveys [20, 23] between 7% and 19% of the population report using acupuncture for various reasons, and studies have shown promising results for its efficacy in adult postoperative and chemotherapy induced nausea and vomiting [23].

In its original form, acupuncture is based on the principles of TCM and involves the insertion of fine needles into the skin along the meridians, providing a means of altering the flow of energy through the body. In a typical treatment, between 4 to 10 points are needled for 10–30 minutes. Needles can be stimulated by manual twirling or with a small electric current, as electroacupuncture (EA). There have been few studies of the physiological effects of acupuncture on the male or female reproductive tract, although for many years acupuncture has been widely used as an adjuvant to ART. Opinion about the effectiveness of acupuncture in women undergoing assisted conception varies considerably. Some regard the traditional Chinese treatment as effective whilst others consider acupuncture as primarily a placebo treatment or even as a treatment that is unscientific and futile.

Several meta-analyses have been published in the recent years in this area [24–28]. Depending on the data included and when the reviews were published, researchers have reached different conclusions about the beneficial effects on acupuncture on women undergoing IVF. The most recent Cochrane review showed no evidence of benefit of acupuncture for improving live birth rate (LBR) regardless of whether acupuncture was performed around the time of oocyte retrieval (OR 0.87, 95% CI 0.59–1.29, two studies, n = 464) or around the day of embryo transfer (or 1.22, 95% CI 0.87–1.70, 8 studies, n = 2505). There was no evidence that acupuncture had any effect on pregnancy or miscarriage rates, or had significant side effects [29]. At the time of writing this chapter, the author is aware of five other studies in this area, and the wisdom of the desperate quest to seek results in this ancient Chinese treatment has been questioned by many [30]. Acupuncture is generally accepted to be painless and has few side effects; although recent studies have shown that serious adverse events can occur [31], albeit rarely. In general, clinicians take the view that adjuvant TCM treatment area harmless placebo. Whilst this may be true for acupuncture treatments, the same cannot be said for herbal therapies, which may contain medical constituents which may have adverse effects on superovulation such as oestrogens. There are however no RCTs examining the use of herbal treatments in the ART [32] and a safe approach would be to avoid the use of herbal treatments during ART cycles.

PSYCHOLOGICAL INTERVENTIONS

Assisted reproductive technology (ART) treatment is stressful. Anxiety and depression have been shown in several studies to be responsible for the relatively high dropout rate observed after the first failed IVF cycle [33] although others have reported that psychological factors were not responsible for IVF cycle cancellation or adverse pregnancy outcomes [34] and psychological interventions in an RCT setting did not appear to improve pregnancy outcome [35]. The psychology of patients undertaking medical treatment is complex and whilst some advocate reducing the burden of the treatment by using a mild treatment strategy and managing patient's expectations and the patient journey per se without undue emphasis on treatment success [33], others advocate more aggressive therapy with emphasis placed on early success to avoid disappointment and despondence [36]. Currently no psychological intervention has been shown to improve clinical pregnancy outcome and the data on the beneficial impact of improved psychological health in the ART context is variable. Good clinical practice advocates that counselling services should be provided for patients undergoing ART [21].

CONCLUSION

It is crucial that IVF practitioners understand that studies that have examined the short and long-term adverse outcomes of adjuvant treatments on the women and their offspring after ART treatment are scarce. Based on Barker's hypothesis of the developmental origins of adult disease and the subsequent studies that have dovetailed this theory, it is now known that the alteration of the periconception environment can adversely impact on development and the subsequent detrimental long-term health outcome on the offspring [37]. The use of adjuvants in assisted reproductive treatment should be deliberated cautiously in conjunction with the patient and their partner prior to their treatment.

The Hippocratic principle of doing no harm is especially pertinent to IVF practitioners in relation to the topic discussed in this chapter. In the practice of reproductive medicine, to be honest with our patients regarding the limits of reproductive science, and at times to adopt a supportive doctoring role rather than instituting non-evidence based interventions can be the right thing to do.

Key points for clinical practice

- Hormones:
  - Growth hormones – the routine use of GH on IVF patients cannot be recommended based on the current evidence.
  - There is no evidence to support the use of androgens and androgen modulating agents in ART cycles.
- Anticoagulants – based on highly heterogeneous and low quality data, peri-implantation LMWH administration during assisted reproduction was associated with a significant improvement in live birth rate compared with placebo or no LMWH [odds ratio (or) 1.77, 95% confidence interval (CI) 1.07–2.90]. Given the poor quality data, the routine use of heparin in ART patient is not justified outside the realms of research.
- Endometrial environment:
  - Endometrial injury – the current evidence suggest that endometrial injury in a previous cycle significantly increased the odds of live birth (or 2.46, 95% CI 1.28–4.72) but not during oocyte retrieval due to a significantly lower clinical pregnancy rate in one study (or 0.30, 95% CI 0.14–0.63).
  - Vasodilators and uterine relaxing agents–there is no good evidence currently to support the routine use of these agents at and around the time of embryo transfer.
- Immune-modulating agents:
  - Steroids–the use of glucocorticoids have not been shown to improve pregnancy outcomes in women undergoing IVF/ICSI although a subgroup analysis suggested that there may be borderline beneficial effect when corticosteroids were used in women undergoing IVF alone rather than IVF/ICSI (or 1.50, 95% CI 1.05–2.13). Treatment should therefore be individualised.
  - Intravenous immunoglobulin and intralipids – there is currently no good evidence for the use of these products in ART, which are expensive and have potentially significant adverse effects.
- Traditional Chinese medicine – there is no evidence that acupuncture or herbal remedies improve reproductive outcome in ART.
- Good clinical practice advocates counselling services to be provided for patients undergoing ART.

REFERENCES

1. Kucuk T, Kozinoglu H, Kaba A. Growth hormone co-treatment within a GnRH agonist long protocol in patients with poor ovarian response: a prospective, randomized, clinical trial. J Assist Reprod Genet 2008; 25:123–127.
2. Mendoza C, Cremades N, Ruiz-Requena E, et al. Relationship between fertilization results after intracytoplasmic sperm injection, and intrafollicular steroid, pituitary hormone and cytokine concentrations. Hum Reprod 1999; 14:628–635.

3. Sugaya S, Suzuki M, Fujita K, et al. Effect of cotreatment with growth hormone on ovarian stimulation in poor responders to in vitro fertilization. Fertil Steril 2003; 79:1251–1253.
4. Tesarik J, Hazout A, Mendoza C. Improvement of delivery and live birth rates after ICSI in women aged >40 years by ovarian co-stimulation with growth hormone. Hum Reprod 2005; 20:2536–2541.
5. Dor J, Seidman DS, Amudai E, et al. Adjuvant growth hormone therapy in poor responders to in-vitro fertilization: a prospective randomized placebo-controlled double-blind study. Hum Reprod 1995; 10:40–43.
6. Eftekhar M, Aflatoonian A, Mohammadian F, et al. Adjuvant growth hormone therapy in antagonist protocol in poor responders undergoing assisted reproductive technology. Arch Gynecol Obstet 2013; 287:1017–10721.
7. Kolibianakis EM, Venetis CA, Diedrich K, et al. Addition of growth hormone to gonadotrophins in ovarian stimulation of poor responders treated by in-vitro fertilization: a systematic review and meta-analysis. Human Reprod Update 2009; 15:613–622.
8. Vendola KA, Zhou J, Adesanya OO, et al. Androgens stimulate early stages of follicular growth in the primate ovary. J Clin Invest 1998; 101:2622–2629.
9. Feigenberg T, Simon A, Ben-Meir A, et al. Role of androgens in the treatment of patients with low ovarian response. Reprod Biomed Online 2009; 19:888–898.
10. Sunkara SK, Pundir J, Khalaf Y. Effect of androgen supplementation or modulation on ovarian stimulation outcome in poor responders: a meta-analysis. Reprod Biomed Online 2011; 22:545–555.
11. Narkwichean A, Maalouf W, Campbell BK, et al. Efficacy of dehydroepiandrosterone to improve ovarian response in women with diminished ovarian reserve: a meta-analysis. Reprod Biol Endocrinol 2013; 11:44.
12. Akhtar MA, Sur S, Raine-Fenning N, et al. Heparin for assisted reproduction. Cochrane Database Syst Rev 2013; 8:CD009452.
13. El-Toukhy T, Sunkara S, Khalaf Y. Local endometrial injury and IVF outcome: a systematic review and meta-analysis. Reprod Biomed Online 2012; 25:345–354.
14. Narvekar SA, Gupta N, Shetty N, et al. Does local endometrial injury in the nontransfer cycle improve the IVF-ET outcome in patients with previous unsuccessful IVF? A randomized controlled pilot study. J Human Reprod Sci 2010; 3:15–19.
15. Nastri CO, Gibreel A, Raine-Fenning N, et al. Endometrial injury in women undergoing assisted reproductive techniques. Cochrane Database Systematic Rev 2012; 7:CD009517.
16. Nardo LG, Granne I, Stewart J; Policy & Practice Committee of the British Fertility Society. Medical adjuncts in IVF: evidence for clinical practice. Human Fertil (Camb) 2009; 12:1–13
17. Cheong Y, Boomsma C, Heijnen C, et al. Uterine secretomics: a window on the maternal–embryo interface. Fertil Steril 2013; 99:1093–1099.
18. Koot YE, Macklon NS. Embryo implantation: biology, evaluation, and enhancement. Curr Opin Obstet Gynecol 2013; 25:274–279.
19. Boomsma CM, Macklon NS. Does glucocorticoid therapy in the peri-implantation period have an impact on IVF outcomes? Curr Opin Obstet Gynecol 2008; 20:249–256.
20. Klein SD, Frei-Erb M, Wolf U. Usage of complementary medicine across Switzerland: results of the Swiss Health Survey 2007. Swiss Med Wkly 2012; 142:w13666.
21. Fields E, Chard J, James D, et al. Fertility (update): summary of NICE guidance. BMJ 2013; 346:f650.
22. IVIg Guideline Development Group of the IVIg Expert Working Group. Clinical guidelines for immunoglobulin use, 2nd edn. London: Department of Health, 2008.
23. NIH Consensus Conference. Acupuncture. JAMA 1998; 1518–1524.
24. Anderson BJ, Haimovici F, Ginsburg ES, et al. In vitro fertilization and acupuncture: clinical efficacy and mechanistic basis. Altern Ther Health Med 2007; 13:38–48.
25. Cheong YC, Hung Yu Ng E, Ledger WL. Acupuncture and assisted conception. Cochrane Database Syst Rev 2008; :CD006920.
26. Manheimer E, van der Windt D, Cheng K, et al. The effects of acupuncture on rates of clinical pregnancy among women undergoing in vitro fertilization: a systematic review and meta-analysis. Human Reprod Update 2013; 19:696–713.
27. Zheng CH, Huang GY, Zhang MM, et al. Effects of acupuncture on pregnancy rates in women undergoing in vitro fertilization: a systematic review and meta-analysis. Fertil Steril 2012; 97:599–611.
28. Manheimer E, Zhang G, Udoff L, et al. Effects of acupuncture on rates of pregnancy and live birth among women undergoing in vitro fertilisation: systematic review and meta-analysis. BMJ 2008; 336:545–549.
29. Cheong YC, Dix S, Hung Yu Ng E, et al. Acupuncture and assisted reproductive technology. Cochrane Database Syst Rev 2013; 7:CD006920.

30. El-Toukhy T, Khalaf Y. A new study of acupuncture in IVF: pointing in the right direction. Reprod Biomed Online 2010; 21:278–279.
31. He W, Zhao X, Li Y, et al. Adverse events following acupuncture: a systematic review of the Chinese literature for the years 1956–2010. J Altern Complement Med 2012; 18:892–901.
32. Cheong Y, Nardo LG, Rutherford T, et al. Acupuncture and herbal medicine in in vitro fertilisation: a review of the evidence for clinical practice. Human Fertil 2010; 13:3–12.
33. Verberg MF, Eijkemans MJ, Heijnen EM, et al. Why do couples drop-out from IVF treatment? A prospective cohort study. Hum Reprod 2008; 23:2050–2055.
34. Lintsen AM, Verhaak CM, Eijkemans MJ, et al. Anxiety and depression have no influence on the cancellation and pregnancy rates of a first IVF or ICSI treatment. Hum Reprod 2009; 24:1092–1098.
35. de Klerk C, Macklon NS, Heijnen EM J, et al. The psychological impact of IVF failure after two or more cycles of IVF with a mild versus standard treatment strategy. Hum Reprod 2007; 22:2554–2558.
36. Flisser E, Copperman AB. Why do couples drop-out from IVF treatment? Hum Reprod 2009; 24:758–759.
37. Barker DJ. Developmental origins of adult health and disease. J Epidemiol Community Health 2004; 58:114–115.

Chapter 13

Kisspeptin, a novel regulator of pituitary gonadotrophins

Waljit S Dhillo, Chioma Izzi-Engbeaya

INTRODUCTION

The kisspeptin gene, *KISS1*, located on chromosome 1, was initially discovered in 1996 and it was found to be a metastasis suppressor gene in malignant melanoma and breast cancer cells [1]. It was named after Hershey's kisses (KI) and its putated function ('SS' for 'suppressor sequence'). However, further work has revealed that its products, named 'kisspeptins', play a vital role in acquiring and maintaining the ability to reproduce in humans and all mammals that have been studied. Kisspeptins primarily control the release of gonadotrophin-releasing hormone (GnRH), with resultant effects on pituitary gonadotrophin and sex hormone production.

KISSPEPTINS, THE KISSPEPTIN RECEPTOR AND KISSPEPTIN NEURONES

The kisspeptins are produced by the cleavage of the 145 amino acid precursor peptide encoded by the *KISS1* gene, and each kisspeptin is named based on the length of its amino acid chain. All kisspeptins have an identical C-terminal 10 amino acid chain, which is required for biological activity. This kisspeptin, called kisspeptin-10, is the smallest kisspeptin [2]. Other kisspeptins include kisspeptin-13, kisspeptin-14, and kisspeptin-52 (in rodents), but the main product of the precursor peptide in humans is kisspeptin-54 (originally called metastin) [3]. The kisspeptins belong to the arginine-phenylalanine (RF) amide peptide hormone family and they activate the G-protein coupled receptor 54 (GPR54) [2], also known as the kisspeptin receptor (KISS1R). The kisspeptin receptor gene (*KISS1R*) is expressed in the hypothalamus, as well as within cortical and subcortical regions [4]. Outside the central nervous system, *KISS1R* expression is found in pituitary gonadotrophs, the placenta, heart, skeletal muscle, kidney and liver [5–7].

Waljit S Dhillo MBBS MRCP PhD, Section of Investigative Medicine, Division of Diabetes, Endocrinology and Metabolism, Imperial College London at Hammersmith Campus, London, UK.

Chioma Izzi-Engbeaya BSc MBBS MRCP, Section of Investigative Medicine, Division of Diabetes, Endocrinology and Metabolism, Imperial College London at Hammersmith Campus, London, UK. Email: c.izzi@imperial.ac.uk (for correspondence)

Using in situ hybridisation and immunocytochemisty, kisspeptin neurones have been identified in the infundibular nucleus in humans and its equivalent in other mammals, [i.e. the arcuate nucleus (ARC)] and the preoptic region [the preoptic area (POA) in humans and large mammals and the anteroventral periventricular nucleus (AVPV) in rodents] [8–11]. There are higher numbers of kisspeptin neurones in the infundibular nucleus (INF)/ARC than in the POA [8]. There is sexual dimorphism in their distribution as evidenced by the fact that kisspeptin neurones have been detected in the POA in women but not in men [9].

Other differences exist between the ARC kisspeptin neurones and the POA/AVPV kisspeptin neurones. ARC kisspeptin neurones (but not the POA/AVPV kisspeptin neurones) co-express neurokinin B (NKB) and dynorphin (DYN) [12]. Both NKB and DYN participate in the control of GnRH secretion, and these specialised kisspeptin-NKB-DYN (KNDY) neurones form an extensive interconnected network [13]. Furthermore, the majority (50-99%) of the kisspeptin neurones in the ARC and preoptic region express the alpha isoform of the oestrogen receptor (ERα) and the progesterone receptor (PR) [10,11,14]. However, only 11–31% of kisspeptin neurones in these regions express the beta isoform of the oestrogen receptor (ERβ)[11,14].

KISSPEPTIN AND GONADOTROPHIN-RELEASING HORMONE

Evidence for the role of kisspeptin in GnRH secretion continues to accumulate. Direct contacts between kisspeptin fibres and GnRH neurones have been demonstrated using electron microscopy [15]. Kisspeptin stimulates GnRH secretion [16] by acting directly on GnRH nerve terminals [17]. Additionally, GnRH neurones express the kisspeptin receptor [18], and GnRH release in response to kisspeptin-10 administration does not occur in mice that lack the kisspeptin receptor [17,18].

Puberty

One of the hallmarks of puberty is activation of the dormant hypothalamus-pituitary-gonadal axis, with commencement of the pattern of regular pulsatile GnRH secretion. Pulsatile GnRH secretion results in pulsatile secretion of the pituitary gonadotrophins [luteinising hormone (LH) and follicle-stimulating hormone (FSH)], which in turn result in gonadal sex steroid production (oestrogens and progesterone from the ovaries in females), gametogenesis and development of secondary sexual characteristics. Both an increase in hypothalamic kisspeptin mRNA and increased sensitivity of the kisspeptin receptor have been noted early in puberty [19]. In ewe lambs, the number of kisspeptin-expressing neurones in the POA increases during the peripubertal period and this is accompanied by the emergence of pulsatile LH secretion [20]. Similarly in ewes, a larger number of kisspeptin cells and almost double the number of kisspeptin-GnRH neurone connections are present in the POA postpubertally compared with prepubertally [21].

In non-human primates, the release of kisspeptin increases throughout pubertal maturation [22], the frequency of kisspeptin pulses increases as puberty advances [23], and this is associated with the pubertal increase in GnRH secretion [22]. Kisspeptin administration to prepubertal female rats results in gonadotrophin secretion, and advances vaginal opening (a cardinal sign of pubertal maturation in rodents) [19]. Similarly, repetitive administration of kisspeptin to prepubertal female lambs increases ovarian steriodogenesis and induces a preovulatory LH surge [20]. Furthermore, the onset of pubertal maturation is delayed in female rats following administration of a *KISS1R* antagonist [24], indicating that kisspeptin stimulation of GnRH neurones is important for the activation of GnRH neurones that occurs at the onset of puberty.

Activating mutations of *KISS1R* [25] and *KISS1* [26] cause precocious puberty. Higher kisspeptin levels have been reported in girls with premature thelarche [27] and central precocious puberty [28]. Conversely, inactivating mutations of *KISS1*, *KISS1R*, the NKB gene (*TAC3*) and the NKB receptor gene (*TAC3R*) result in isolated hypogonadotrophic hypogonadism, and patients with these mutations either do not go through puberty (without the administration of exogenous hormones) or have delayed puberty [26,29–31]. Therefore, it appears that normal kisspeptin release and action is required for the appropriate timing, onset and progression of puberty.

However, in contrast to the above reports, a research group that generated two types of knockout female mice (the first of which lacked kisspeptin-expressing cells and the second lacked kisspeptin receptor expression) found that in both types of mice puberty onset and progression was no different to wild-type controls except that the mass of the ovaries in the knockout mice was smaller [32]. Furthermore, both types of knockout mice were fertile and all had offspring after mating. It is possible that the knockout models were not complete, since around 3% of the normal number of kisspeptin neurones were found in the knockout mice [32] and a subsequent study that used similar knockout mice demonstrated that minute amounts of kisspeptin are sufficient for pubertal development to occur with subsequent fertility [33]. An alternative explanation is that biological compensation may occur if kisspeptin or kisspeptin neurones are absent during early embryological development, which enable puberty to occur and therefore maintain fertility.

Adulthood

Insights into the role of kisspeptin in regulating pituitary gonadotrophin release in pre-menopausal females have been provided by a number of clinical studies. Following on from animal studies which demonstrated that kisspeptin potently stimulated GnRH-mediated LH and FSH secretion, the first human study showed that peripheral intravenous administration of kisspeptin-54 at a dose of 2 pmol/kg/min resulted in a significant increase in LH, FSH and testosterone levels in men [34]. In women, a single subcutaneous injection of kisspeptin-54 (at a dose of 0.3 or 0.6 nmol/kg) not only increased LH levels, but it also increased LH pulsatility [35]. Chronic subcutaneous administration of kisspeptin-54 (6.4 nmol/kg twice daily for 7 days during the follicular phase of the menstrual cycle) advanced the onset of the luteal phase and shortens the length of the menstrual cycle by 2 days [36]. These studies confirm that kisspeptin stimulates gonadotrophin release in vivo in humans.

Acute kisspeptin-54 administration increased circulating levels of LH during each phase of the menstrual cycle but its effect was greatest during the pre-ovulatory phase (i.e. 15–16 days before the next predicted period) [37]. Kisspeptin-10 also stimulates LH secretion in the pre-ovulatory and luteal phases of the menstrual cycle but it has a less marked effect in the follicular phase [38]. Therefore, in women the sensitivity to kisspeptin varies during different phases of the menstrual cycle, with the lowest sensitivity occurring during the follicular phase.

There is sexual dimorphism in the response to kisspeptin. Kisspeptin-10 administration to men in doses as low as 1.0 nmol/kg produces elevations in serum LH and FSH levels [39]. However, intravenous or subcutaneous administration of kisspeptin-10 to women in doses up to 10 nmol/kg does not change serum gonadotrophin levels during the follicular phase, but administration of 10 nmol/kg of kisspeptin-10 during the pre-ovulatory phase produces an elevation in serum gonadotrophin levels [39]. Therefore, women appear to be less sensitive to kisspeptin-10 compared to men, and women may be more sensitive to kisspeptin-54 than kisspeptin-10. Furthermore, in rodents, men and women, kisspeptin produces greater elevations in LH levels than FSH levels [16,34,37].

Women with functional hypothalamic amenorrhoea (i.e. absence of menstruation due to abnormal signalling between the hypothalamus and pituitary gland with structurally normal hypothalamus and pituitary) have abnormal reproductive hormone profiles consisting of low serum gonadotrophin and oestradiol levels (i.e. hypogonadotrophic hypogonadism). Administration of 6.4 nmol/kg kisspeptin-54 acutely stimulates gonadotrophin secretion and the elevations in LH levels produced is four times greater than that seen in healthy women in the follicular phase of the menstrual cycle [40]. However, after 2 weeks of chronic administration of kisspeptin-54 to women with hypothalamic amenorrhoea (at a dose of 6.4 nmol/kg twice a day) only very small elevations in gonadotrophins were elicited post-kisspeptin injection but the response to GnRH injections was preserved [40]. Thus, women with functional hypothalamic amenorrhoea are more sensitive to kisspeptin-54 than healthy women and desensitisation to kisspeptin stimulation (but not GnRH) occurs after 2 weeks of twice daily high dose kisspeptin-54 injections (a phenomenon known as tachyphylaxis). This may be due to downregulation of the kisspeptin receptor in response to chronic stimulation with high doses of kisspeptin. When kisspeptin-54 was administered to women with hypothalamic amenorrhoea at a dose of 6.4 nmol/kg twice weekly for 8 weeks, partial desensitisation occurred after about 2 weeks and the LH elevation in response to kisspeptin did not diminish further [41]. However, the FSH response was much lower than the LH response and menstrual cyclicity was not restored [41]. Further work has demonstrated that in women with hypothalamic amenorrhoea desensitisation is dose-dependent as continuous infusions of kisspeptin-54 (at doses ranging from 0.01–1.00 nmol/kg/h) for 8 hours temporarily increase LH pulsatility with no desensitisation at lower doses but desensitisation occurring after about 6 hours with the highest dose [42].

It is likely that the feedback effects of oestrogens on gonadotrophin secretion are mediated by kisspeptin. Throughout most of the menstrual cycle oestrogens have a negative feedback effect on gondotrophin secretion (i.e. they suppress gonadotrophin secretion). However, mid-cycle, a change occurs and oestrogens temporarily exert a positive feedback effect on gonadotrophin secretion, which leads to the pre-ovulatory LH surge that is essential for fertility. Adult female rodents that have been given an ERα antagonist do not have a pre-ovulatory LH surge, do not ovulate, and have a blunted LH response to kisspeptin-10 administration [43]. Ovariectomised, oestrogen-replaced mice that lack functional neuronal ERα (due to a null mutation) have normal basal LH levels but do not have pre-ovulatory LH peaks and are infertile [44]. Therefore, signalling via ERα is required for the positive feedback effect of oestrogen that produces the pre-ovulatory LH surge.

GnRH neurones express ERβ but do not express ERα [45], while both the ARC and the AVPV kisspeptin neurones express ERα [10,11,14]. In female mice, oestrogen deficiency (caused by ovariectomy) results in decreased kisspeptin gene (Kiss1) expression in the AVPV and increased Kiss1 expression in the ARC [14, 46]. Oestrogen replacement in these animals causes the reverse, i.e. increased Kiss1 expression in the AVPV and decreased Kiss1 expression in the ARC [14]. Additionally, ERα is required for the oestrogen-induced suppression of kisspeptin gene expression in the ARC [14]. These studies indicate that the two populations of kisspeptin neurones respond differently to oestrogens via ERα. The positive feedback of oestrogen on AVPV kisspeptin neurones results in increased GnRH secretion and resulting increased LH secretion. The negative feedback effect of oestrogens on ARC kisspeptin neurones results in decreased kisspeptin secretion and consequently GnRH, and LH secretion is also decreased.

Lactation and hyperprolactinaemia

During lactation prolactin levels are elevated and prolactin secretion is stimulated by suckling. Ovulation and menstrual cyclicity cease for some time during lactation, with associated reduced LH pulsatile secretion likely secondary to inhibition of GnRH secretion [47]. In rats, very low levels of *Kiss1* mRNA (in both the ARC and AVPV) are detected during lactation [47, 48]. Additionally, reduced kisspeptin levels are found in the ARC neurones whilst increased kisspeptin levels are found within the neurones of the AVPV [49]. This indicates that both the manufacture and release (i.e. secretion) of kisspeptin is affected by lactation, and there may be different effects on the different population of kisspeptin neurones.

In keeping with the theory that during lactation kisspeptin secretion is inhibited with subsequent suppression of GnRH secretion, administration of kisspeptin-54 into the central nervous system of rats during lactation results in increased LH secretion [48]. Additionally, increased ARC kisspeptin is found when pulsatile LH secretion resumes after lactation ceases due to removal of rat pups [47].

Hyperprolactinaemia in the non-lactating female (and in men) causes hypogonadotrophic hypogonadism. Less than 15% of GnRH neurones express prolactin receptors whilst kisspeptin neurones possess significant numbers of prolactin receptors [50]. Therefore, prolactin-induced GnRH suppression is likely to occur indirectly via kisspeptin inhibition. In a study where prolactin was continuously infused into female mice (to produce and maintain hyperprolactinaemia), the mice had irregular or absent cycles, and once daily injection of kisspeptin-10 restored LH secretion, menstrual cyclicity and ovulation despite on-going prolactin infusion [51]. Furthermore, in this study constant infusion of prolactin resulted in reduced kisspeptin protein in the ARC and AVPV of the mice [51]. Additional information about the relationship between prolactin and kisspeptin was provided by a study in rats in which kisspeptin-10 was found to increase prolactin secretion (via inhibition of hypothalamic dopamine release) in a dose-dependent manner in oestradiol-treated ovariectomised rats (and male rats) but had no effect on oil-treated ovariectomised rats [52]. Thus, kisspeptin may stimulate prolactin secretion while prolactin may exert a negative feedback effect on kisspeptin release.

Undernutrition and overnutrition

Negative energy balance [53] and obesity [54] are both known to cause hypogonadotrophic hypogonadism. Both these states may produce suppression of gonadotrophin secretion via inhibition of kisspeptin signalling. Fasting causes a reduction in hypothalamic *Kiss1* mRNA and peripheral LH levels in pubertal and adult rats [55,56]. In female rats whose pubertal development was arrested by chronic undernutrition, kisspeptin-10 administration caused pubertal progression to occur and produced elevations of gonadotrophins and oestrogens [55]. Similarly, in women with underweight-induced hypogonadotrophic hypogonadism, kisspeptin-54 administration resulted in elevated gonadotropin and oestrogen levels [40, 41].

Leptin is a hormone that is secreted by adipocytes (fat cells), and its secretion is proportional to the individual's fat mass. Leptin provides the brain with information about the individual's nutritional status, and it reduces appetite. As fat mass increases, leptin levels increase. However, in obesity a state of central leptin resistance occurs. In prepubertal rats that receive different food regimens there is a positive correlation between circulating leptin levels and hypothalamic *Kiss1* and kisspeptin receptor gene (*Kiss1r*) mRNA levels [57]. Central administration of kisspeptin-10 to leptin resistant (overfed) and leptin deficient (underfed) mice (which have hypogonadotrophic hypogonadism) produced elevations in gonadotrophin levels [19,57]. Kisspeptin neurones express the leptin receptor and leptin does not act directly on GnRH neurones [58]. Therefore, kisspeptin and leptin may provide a link between nutritional status and reproductive function.

Compared with normal mice, congenitally leptin deficient (ob/ob) mice are obese, have lower *Kiss1* mRNA levels in the ARC [59,60], fewer kisspeptin-immunoreactive cells in the AVPV [60], and exhibit hypogonadotrophic hypogondadism [59]. Infusion of leptin to ob/ob mice increased *Kiss1* expression in the ARC [59]. Similarly, diet-induced obese female mice (i.e. a mouse model of leptin resistance) have markedly reduced *Kiss1* mRNA in both the ARC and AVPV, with fewer kisspeptin-expressing cells detected in the AVPV [60]. Female mice lacking functional leptin receptors (i.e. leptin resistant mice) do not have the increase in kisspeptin neurone activation produced by the positive feedback of pre-ovulatory surge oestradiol levels, and consequently do not generate preovulatory GnRH and LH surges [60].

These animal data suggest that leptin regulates GnRH and therefore gonadotrophin secretion by stimulating kisspeptin production, with reduced kisspeptin expression (and subsequent hypogonadotrophic hypogonadism) in leptin deficient and leptin resistant conditions. However recent work suggests that leptin may not directly stimulate kisspeptin neurones (with resultant GnRH neurone stimulation) as selective genetic deletion of the leptin receptor from hypothalamic kisspeptin neurones in mice did not result in abnormal pubertal development or infertility [61]. However, bilateral lesions of the ventral premammillary nucleus (PMV; an area of the brain not known to contain kisspeptin neurones) in congenitally leptin deficient (ob/ob) mice blunted the ability of exogenous leptin to induce puberty [61]. Additionally, selective re-expression of the leptin receptor gene in kisspeptin neurones in mice with generalised leptin receptor deficiency did not result in pubertal development and the mice were infertile [62].

In humans there is limited data available about the relationship between body weight, leptin and kisspeptin. In one report, higher circulating kisspeptin levels were found in obese prepubertal girls and in these girls kisspeptin levels were found to correlate with leptin levels [28]. Administration of recombinant leptin to women with hypothalamic amenorrhoea due to low body weight or strenuous exercise restores LH pulsatility (accompanied by resumption of ovulatory menstrual cycles in some of the women who received leptin) [53]. Further work is required to clearly define the relationship between leptin and kisspeptin in humans.

Postmenopausal women

The menopause is characterised by ovarian failure and primary hypogonadism, i.e. extremely low oestrogen (and progesterone) levels and significantly elevated pituitary gonadotropin levels. When the hypothalami of premenopausal women and postmenopausal women were compared, kisspeptin neurones were found predominantly in the infundibular nucleus in both groups of women [8]. However, compared with the premenopausal women, the postmenopausal women had much greater numbers of kisspeptin neurones, their kisspeptin neurones were hypertrophied, and their neurones had double the amount of *KISS1* mRNA [8]. Similar changes were found in the hypothalami of young ovariectomised monkeys, but kisspeptin gene expression was reduced to almost undetectable levels in young ovariectomised monkeys that had received oestrogen (or combined oestrogen and progesterone) replacement [8]. Therefore, the elevation in serum gonadotrophins found in postmenopausal females is likely to be a consequence of the absence of the negative feedback effect of oestrogens on kisspeptin, which then results in increased kisspeptin (and subsequent GnRH and gonadotrophin) production.

KISSPEPTIN AND THE ANTERIOR PITUITARY

Although most studies have demonstrated that kisspeptin modulates gonadotrophin secretion indirectly via its effects on GnRH, there is also evidence that kisspeptin can act directly on pituitary gonadotrophs. The genes for both kisspeptin and its receptor are expressed in pituitary gonadotrophs [2, 7], and in vitro exposure of mammalian pituitary cells and tissue to kisspeptin-10 results in dose-dependent LH release [63]. Treatment with kisspeptin-10 significantly increased expression of LH and FSH in mice pituitary cultures, but expression of the GnRH receptor was not increased [64]. Furthermore, the expression of the kisspeptin receptor in the pituitary of female mice was induced by oestradiol during the pre-ovulatory LH-surge [64]. Therefore, kisspeptin can act directly on pituitary gonadotropes to stimulate LH and FSH gene expression and protein secretion, and the positive feedback of oestrogen which produces the LH surge may act not only on the hypothalamus but also act directly on the pituitary. However, further research is required to determine the physiological roles (if any) of any direct kisspeptin-pituitary interaction(s).

The effect of oestrogen on kisspeptin expression in the pituitary is similar to its effect in the hypothalamus. Administration of a selective ERα antagonist to ovariectomised rats caused about a five-fold increase in pituitary *Kiss1* expression, but administration of a selective ERβ antagonist had no effect [7]. Interestingly, in the same study, administration of a selective ERβ antagonist alone, a selective ERβ antagonist alone, and a combination of both antagonists resulted in a decrease in *Kiss1r* expression in the pituitary [7]. The hormonal regulation of pituitary gonadotrophins in adult females, mediated by kisspeptin, is illustrated in **Figure 13.1**.

POTENTIAL CLINICAL USES OF KISSPEPTIN

Given the actions of kisspeptin in the regulation of pituitary gonadotrophins, there are a number of potential therapeutic uses for kisspeptin. Kisspeptin administration has been shown to stimulate gonadotrophin secretion with resultant increased sex hormone release in mice with hyperprolactinaemia-induced ovarian acyclicity [51], healthy women [35], women with hypothalamic amenorrhoea [42], healthy men [34], obese men with type 2 diabetes and hypogonadism [65], and people with neurokinin B receptor mutations [66]. Furthermore, kisspeptin administration has been shown to reset the GnRH pulse generator in men [67]. Therefore, kisspeptin could be used to treat anovulatory disorders and restore fertility to women by restoring endogenous GnRH pulsatility.

Women who require infertility treatment in the form of assisted conception currently receive protocols consisting of the administration of a GnRH agonist for several days (to desensitise the pituitary) followed by gonadotrophin administration (to stimulate follicular

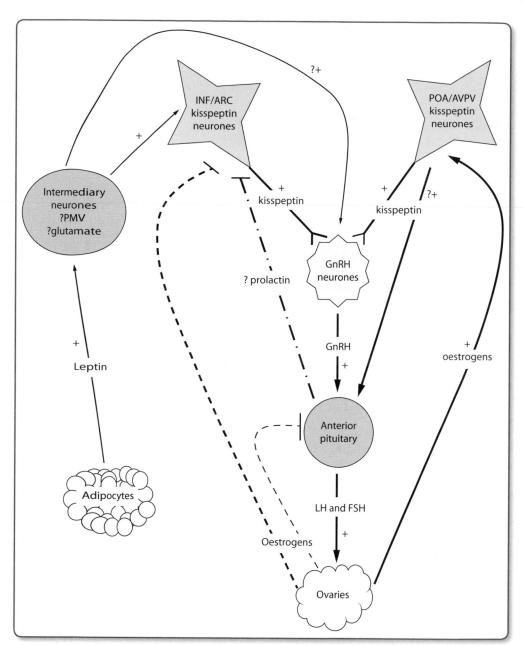

Figure 13.1 Regulation of pituitary gonadotrophins in adult females. Kisspeptin neurones stimulate GnRH neurones to secrete GnRH, which in turn stimulates anterior pituitary gonadotrophs to release LH and FSH. The gonadotrophins stimulate the ovaries to secrete oestrogens. Kisspeptin may also stimulate the pituitary gonadotrophs directly to release gonadotrophins, but in vivo this does not play a major role in gonadotropin secretion. Oestrogens inhibit secretion of kisspeptin from the INF/ARC neurones and inhibit pituitary gonadotrophin secretion. However in the pre-ovulatory phase of the menstrual cycle, oestrogens stimulate POA/AVPV kisspeptin neurones to release kisspeptin. Prolactin from the anterior pituitary may inhibit kisspeptin secretion. Inhibition of kisspeptin secretion leads to a reduction in GnRH and consequent reduction in gonadotrophin secretion. Leptin, secreted by adipocytes, may stimulate kisspeptin secretion via intermediary neurones, but its role in kisspeptin-mediated gonadotrophin secretion has not yet been fully elucidated. INF/ARC, infundibular nucleus/arcuate nucleus; POA/AVPV, preoptic area/anteroventral periventricular nucleus; PMV, ventral premammillary nucleus.

growth), with subsequent administration of **human chorionic gonadotropin** (hCG) (to stimulate oocyte maturation) prior to egg collection. In other regimes GnRH antagonists are used (instead of GnRH agonists) to switch off endogenous gonadotrophin secretion. However, assisted conception cycles using these regimes may be complicated by ovarian hyperstimulation syndrome (OHSS) (a systemic disease caused by the release of vasoactive substances released by hyperstimulated ovaries), with 3–8% of cycles complicated by moderate or severe OHSS [68]. Severe OHSS requires inpatient admission and specialist management, and may result in multiorgan dysfunction or death. The cause of OHSS is the use of hCG which has a prolonged LH-like action. Since kisspeptin stimulates endogenous gonadotrophin release it may be a more physiological alternative to hCG for stimulation of follicular maturation, and compared with hCG its use may therefore result in a lower risk of OHSS. Studies are currently underway to investigate the use of kisspeptin as a trigger for oocyte maturation in assisted conception, and the results of these studies are awaited.

Kisspeptin receptor antagonism results in reduced GnRH and LH secretion. This offers a target for development of contraceptive agents, or for development of hormone deprivation therapies for hormone-sensitive cancers (such as breast cancer and prostate cancer) and hormone-dependent reproductive disorders like central precocious puberty. A kisspeptin receptor antagonist (Peptide 234, a kisspeptin-10 analogue) has already been shown to inhibit kisspeptin-10 stimulation of GnRH neurone firing in the brains of mice, GnRH release in pubertal female monkeys and rats, and inhibit LH pulses in ovariectomised ewes [69]. Since high-doses of kisspeptin can produce tachyphylaxis in certain circumstances [40], this may provide an alternative means of suppressing the hormonal reproductive axis. Recently, a phase 1 trial involving men aged 50–78 years, reported that a single 0.1 mg subcutaneous bolus of a kisspeptin receptor analogue (TAK-448) produced a surge in gonadotropin levels (and a slight increase in testosterone) 12 hours later, but a continuous subcutaneous infusion of the analogue for 13 days resulted in complete testosterone suppression [70].

CONCLUSION

Although kisspeptin was discovered less than two decades ago, a substantial body of evidence about its actions and functions has accumulated. This has provided new insights into the control of pituitary gonadotrophins and reproductive physiology. Manipulation of kisspeptin signalling can be used to develop new treatments for reproductive disorders and sex hormone-deprivation therapies. Further work is required as so many questions remain unanswered, and it will be interesting to see what future research reveals.

Key points for clinical practice

- Kisspeptin plays a pivotal role in puberty and maintenance normal reproductive function, by regulating pituitary gonadotrophin secretion via GnRH stimulation.
- Kisspeptin could be used to stimulate ovulation and may prove to be useful in treating certain reproductive disorders.
- Kisspeptin receptor antagonists and kisspeptin analogues are being investigated in order to develop agents that suppress reproductive hormone secretion, which may be used as contraceptive agents and/or as part of the treatment of sex hormone-sensitive cancers.

REFERENCES

1. Lee JH, Miele ME, Hicks DJ, et al. KISS-1, a novel human malignant melanoma metastasis-suppressor gene. J Natl Cancer Inst 1996; 88:1731–1737.
2. Kotani M, Detheux M, Vandenboagaerde A, et al. The metastasis suppressor gene KISS-1 encodes kisspeptins, the natural ligands of the orphan G protein-coupled receptor GPR54. J Biol Chem 2001; 276:34631–34636.
3. Ohtaki T, Shintanu Y, Honda S, et al. Metastasis suppressor gene KISS-1 encodes peptide ligand of a G-protein-coupled receptor. Nature 2001; 411:613–617.
4. Lee DK, Nguyen T, O'Neill GP, et al. Discovery of a receptor related to the galanin receptors. FEBS Lett 1999; 446:103–107.
5. Muir AI, Chamberlain L, Elshourbagy NA, et al. AXOR12, a novel human G protein-coupled receptor, activated by the peptide KiSS-1. J Biol Chem 2001; 276:28969–28975.
6. Clements MK, McDonald TP, Wang R, et al. FMRFamide-Related neuropeptides are agonists of the orphan G-protein-coupled receptor GPR54. Biochem Biophys Res Commun 2001; 284:1189–1193.
7. Richard N, Galmiche G, Corvaisier S, et al. KiSS-1 and GPR54 genes are co-expressed in rat gonadotrophs and differentially regulated in vivo by oestradiol and gonadotrophin-releasing hormone. J Neuroendocrinol 2008; 29:381–393.
8. Rometo AM, Krajewaski SJ, Voytko ML, et al. Hypertrophy and increased kisspeptin gene expression in the hypothalamic infundibular nucleus of postmenopausal women and ovariectomized monkeys. J Clin Endocrinol Metab 2007; 92:2744–2750.
9. Hrabovszky E, Ciofi P, Vida B, et al. The kisspeptin system of the human hypothalamus: sexual dimorphism and relationship with gonadotrophin-releasing hormone and neurokinin B neurons. Eur J Neurosci 2010; 31:1984–1998.
10. Adachi S, Yamada S, Takatsu Y, et al. Involvement of anteroventricular periventricular metastin/kisspeptin neurons in estrogen positive feedback action on luteinizing hormone release in rats. J Reprod Dev 2007; 53:367–378.
11. Smith JT, Popa SM, Clifton DK, et al. KISS1 neurons in the forebrain as central processors for generating the preovulatory luteinizing hormone surge. J Neurosci 2006; 26:6687–6694.
12. Goodman RL, Lehman MN, Smith JT, et al. Kisspeptin neurons in the arcuate nucleus of the ewe express both dynorphin A and neurokinin B. Endocrinol 2007; 148:5752–5760.
13. Krajewski SJ, Burke MC, Anderson MJ, et al. Forebrain projections of arcuate neurokinin B neurons demonstrated by anterograde tract-tracing and monosodium glutamate lesions in the rat. Neurosci 2010; 166:680–697.
14. Smith JT, Cunningham MJ, Rissman EF, et al. Regulation of Kiss1 gene expression in the brain of the female mouse. Endocrinology 2005; 146:3686–3692.
15. Kalló I, Vida B, Deli L, et al. Co-localisation of kisspeptin with galanin or neurokinin B in afferents to mouse GnRH neurones. J Neuroendocrinol 2012; 24:464–476.
16. Thompson EL, Patterson M, Murphy KG, et al. Central and peripheral administration of kisspeptin-10 stimulates the hypothalamic-pituitary-gonadal axis. J Neuroendocrinol 2004; 16:850–858.
17. d'Anglemont de Tassigny X, Fagg LA, Carlton MBL, et al. Kisspeptin can stimulate gonadotropin-releasing hormone (GnRH) release by a direct action at GnRH nerve terminals. Endocrinology 2008; 149:3926–3932.
18. Messager S, Chatzidaki EE, Ma D, et al. Kisspeptin directly stimulates gonadotropin-releasing hormone release via G protein-coupled receptor 54. Proc Natl Acad Sci USA 2005; 102:1761–1766.
19. Navarro VM, Fernandez-Fernandez R, Castellano JM, et al. Advanced vaginal opening and precocious activation of the reproductive axis by KiSS-1 peptide, the endogenous ligand of GPR54. J Physiol 2004; 561:379–386.
20. Redmond JS, Macedo GG, Velez LC, et al. Kisspeptin activates the hypothalamic-adenohypophyseal-gonadal axis in prepubertal lambs. Reproduction 2011; 141:541–548.
21. Nestor CC, Briscoe AMS, Davis SM, et al. Evidence of role for kisspeptin and neurokinin B in puberty of female sheep. Endocrinology 2012; 153:2756–2765.
22. Keen KL, Wegner FH, Bloom SR, et al. An increase in kisspeptin-54 release occurs with the pubertal increase in luteinizing hormone-releasing hormone-1 release in the stalk median eminence of female rhesus monkeys in vivo. Endocrinology 2008; 149:4151–4157.
23. Guerriero KA, Keen KL, Terasawa E. Developmental increase in kisspeptin-54 release in vivo is independent of the pubertal increase in estradiol in female rhesus monkeys (Macaca mulatta). Endocrinology 2012; 153:1887–1897.

24. Pineda R, Garcia-Galiano D, Roseweir A, et al. Critical roles of kisspeptins in female puberty and preovulatory gonadotropin surges as revealed by a novel antagonist. Endocrinology 2010; 151:722–730.

25. Teles MG, Bianco SDC, Brito VN, et al. A GPR54-activating mutation in a patient with central precocious puberty. N Engl J Med 2008; 358:709–715.

26. Silveira LG, Noel SD, Silveira-Neto AP, et al. Mutations of the KISS1 gene in disorders of puberty. J Clin Endocrinol Metab 2010; 95:2276–2280.

27. Akinci A, Cetin D, Ilhan N. Plasma kisspeptin level in girls with premature thelarche. J Clin Res Pediatr Endocrinol 2012; 4:61–65.

28. Pita J, Barrios V, Gavela-Perez T, et al. Circulating kisspeptin levels exhibit sexual dimorphism in adults, are increased in obese prepubertal girls and do not suffer modifications in girls with idiopathic central precocious puberty. Peptides 2011; 32:1781–1786.

29. de Roux N, Genin E, Carel JC, et al. Hypogonadotropic hypogonadism due to loss of function of the KiSS1-derived peptide receptor GPR54. Proc Natl Acad Sci USA 2003; 100:10972–10976.

30. Topaloglu AK, Reimann F, Guclu M, et al. TAC3 and TACR3 mutations in familial hypogonadotropic hypogonadism reveal a key role for Neurokinin B in the central control of reproduction. Nat Genet 2009; 41:354–358.

31. Topaloglu AK, Tello JA, Kotan LD, et al. Inactivating KISS1 mutation and hypogonadotropic hypogonadism. N Engl J Med 2012; 366:629–635.

32. Mayer C, Boehm U. Female reproductive maturation in the absence of kisspeptin/GPR54 signalling. Nat Neurosc 2011; 14:704–710.

33. Popa SM, Moriyama RM, Caligioni CS, et al. Redundancy in KISS1 expression safeguards reproduction in the mouse. Endocrinology 2013; 154:2784–2784.

34. Dhillo WS, Chaudhri OB, Patterson M, et al. Kisspeptin-54 stimulates the hypothalamic-pituitary gonadal axis in human males. J Clin Endocrinol Metab 2005; 90:6609–6615.

35. Jayasena CN, Comninos AN, Veldhuis JD, et al. A single injection of kisspeptin-54 temporarily increases luteinizing hormone pulsatility in healthy women. Clin Endocrinol (Oxf) 2013; 79:558–563..

36. Jayasena CN, Comninos AN, Nijher GM, et al. Twice-daily subcutaneous injection of kisspeptin-54 does not abolish menstrual cyclicity in healthy female volunteers. J Clin Endocrinol Metab 2013; 98:4464–4474.

37. Dhillo WS, Chaudhri OB, Thompson EL, et al. Kisspeptin-54 stimulates gonadotropin release most potently during the preovulatory phase of the menstrual cycle in women. J Clin Endocrinol Metab 2007; 92:3958–3966.

38. Chan YM, Butler JP, Sidhoum VF, et al. Kisspeptin administration to women: A window into endogenous kisspeptin secretion and GnRH responsiveness across the menstrual cycle. J Clin Endocrinol Metab 2012; 97:E1458–E1467.

39. Jayasena CN, Nijher GMK, Comninos AN, et al. The effects of kisspeptin-10 on reproductive hormone release show sexual dimorphism in humans. J Clin Endocrinol Metab 2011; 96:E1963–E1972.

40. Jayasena CN, Nijher GMK, Chaudhri OB, et al. Subcutaneous injection of kisspeptin-54 acutely stimulates gonadotropin secretion in women with hypothalamic amenorrhea, but chronic administration causes tachyphylaxis. J Clin Endocrinol Metab 2009; 94:4315–4323.

41. Jayasena CN, Nijher GMK, Abbara A, et al. Twice-weekly administration of kisspeptin-54 for 8 weeks stimulates release of reproductive hormones in women with hypothalamic amenorrhea. Clin Pharmacol Ther 2010; 88:840–847.

42. Jayasena CN, Abbara A, Veldhuis JD, et al. Increasing LH pulsatility in women with hypothalamic amenorrhea using intravenous infusion of kisspeptin-54. J Clin Endocrinol Metab 2013; in prep.

43. Roa J, Vigo E, Castellano JM, et al. Opposite roles of estrogen receptor (ER)-alpha and ERbeta in the modulation of luteinizing hormone responses to kisspeptin in the female rat: implications for the generation of the preovulatory surge. Endocrinology 2008; 149:1627–1637.

44. Wintermantel TM, Campbell RE, Porteous R, et al. Definition of estrogen receptor pathway critical for estrogen positive feedback to gonadotropin-releasing hormone neurons and fertility. Neuron 2006; 52:271–280.

45. Hrabovszky E, Shughrue PJ, Merchenthaler I, et al. Detection of estrogen receptor-beta messenger ribonucleic acid and 125I-estrogen binding sites in luteinizing hormone-releasing hormone neurons of the rat brain. Endocrinology 2000; 141:3506–3509.

46. Kauffann AS, Navarro VM, Kim J, et al. Sex differences in the regulation of KISS1/NKB neurons in juvenile mice: implications for the timing of puberty. Am J Physiol Endocrinol Metab 2009; 297:E1212–E1221.

47. Xu J, Kirigiti MA, Grove KL, et al. Regulation of food intake and gonadotropin-releasing hormone/luteinizing hormone during lactation: role of insulin and leptin. Endocrinology 2009; 150:4231–4240.

48. Yamada S, Uenoyama Y, Kinoshita M, et al. Inhibition of metastin (kisspeptin-54)-GPR54 signalling in the arcuate nucleus–median eminence region during lactation in rats. Endocrinology 2007; 148:2226–2232.
49. True C, Kirigiti M, Ciofi P, et al. Characterisation of arcuate nucleus kisspeptin/neurokinin N neuronal projections and regulation during lactation in the rat. J Neuroendocrinol 2011; 23:52–64.
50. Kokay IC, Petersen SL, Grattan DR. Identification of prolactin-sensitive GABA and kisspeptin neurons in regions of the rat hypothalamus involved in the control of fertility. Endocrinology 2011; 152:526–535.
51. Sonigo C, Bouilly J, Carre N, et al. Hyperprolactinemia-induced ovarian acyclicity is reversed by kisspeptin administration. J Clin Invest 2012; 122:3791–3795.
52. Szawka RE, Riberiro AB, Leite CM, et al. Kisspeptin regulates prolactin release through hypothalamic dopaminergic neurons. Endocrinology 2010; 151:3247–3257.
53. Welt CK, Chan JL, Bullen J, et al. Recombinant human leptin in women with hypothalamic amenorrhea. N Engl J Med 2004; 351:987–997.
54. Loret de Mola JR. Obesity and its relationship to infertility in men and women. Obst Gynecol Clin North Am 2009; 36:333–346.
55. Castellano JM, Navarro VM, Fernandez-Fernandez R, et al. Changes in hypothalamic KiSS-1 system and restoration of pubertal activation of the reproductive axis by kisspeptin in undernutrition. Endocrinology 2005; 146:3917–3925.
56. Kalamatianos T, Grimshaw SE, Poorun R, et al. Fasting reduces KiSS-1 expression in the anteroventral periventricular nucleus (AVPV): effects of fasting on the expression of KiSS-1 and neuropeptide Y in the AVPV or arcuate nucleus of female rats. J Neuroendocrinol 2008; 20:1089–1097.
57. Castellano JM, Bentsen AH, Sanchez-Garrido MA, et al. Early metabolic programming of puberty onset: impact of changes in postnatal feeding and rearing conditions on the timing of puberty and development of the hypothalamic kisspeptin system. Endocrinology 2011; 152:3396–3408.
58. Quennell JH, Mulligan AC, Tups A, et al. Leptin indirectly regulates gonadotropin-releasing hormone neuronal function. Endocrinology 2009; 150:2805–2812.
59. Smith JT, Acohido BV, Clifton DK, et al. KiSS-1 neurones are direct targets for leptin in the ob/ob mouse. J Neuroendocrinol 2006b; 18:298–303.
60. Quennell JH, Howell CS, Roa J, et al. Leptin deficiency and diet-induced obesity reduce hypothalamic kisspeptin expression in mice. Endocrinology 2011; 152:1541–1550.
61. Donato J Jr, Cravo RM, Frazao R, et al. Leptin's effect on puberty in mice is relayed by the ventral premammillary nucleus and does not require signalling in Kiss1 neurons. J Clin Invest 2011; 121:355–368.
62. Cravo RM, Frazao R, Perello M, et al. Leptin signalling in Kiss1 neurons arises after pubertal development. PLoS One 2013; 8:e58698.
63. Navarro VM, Castellano JM, Fernandez-Fernandez R, et al. Characterization of the potent luteinizing hormone-releasing activity of KiSS-1 peptide, the natural ligand of GPR54. Endocrinology 2005; 146:156–163.
64. Witham EA, Meadows JD, Hoffmann HM, et al. Kisspeptin regulates gonadotropin genes via immediate early gene induction in pituitary gonadotropes. Mol Endocrinol 2013; 27:1283–1294.
65. George JT, Veldhuis JD, Tena-Sempere M, et al. Exploring the pathophysiology of hypogonadism in men with type 2 diabetes: Kisspeptin-10 stimulates serum testosterone and LH secretion in men with type 2 diabetes and mild biochemical hypogonadism. Clin Endocrinol 2013; 79:100–104.
66. Young J, George JT, Tello JA, et al. Kisspeptin restores pulsatile LH secretion in patients with neurokinin B signalling deficiencies: physiological, pathophysiological and therapeutic implications. Neuroendocrinology 2013; 97(2):193–202.
67. Chan YM, Butler JP, Pinnell NE, et al. Kisspeptin resets the hypothalamic GnRH clock in men. J Clin Endocrinol Metab 2011; 96:E908–E915.
68. Royal College of Obstetricians and Gynaecologists (RCOG). The Management of ovarian hyperstimulation syndrome green-top, Guideline No. 5. London; RCOG, 2006.
69. Roseweir AK, Kauffman AS, Smith JT, et al. Discovery of potent kisspeptin antagonists delineate physiological mechanisms of gonadotropin regulation. J Neurosci 2009; 29:3920–3929.
70. MacLean B, Matsui H, Suri A, et al. Investigational kisspeptin/GPR54 agonist peptide analog, TAK-448, given as single-dose then 13-day continuous subcutaneous infusion, stimulates then suppresses the LH-testosterone axis in healthy male volunteers. Poster session presented at: The Endocrine Society's 95th Annual Meeting and Expo; San Francisco, 2013. Poster number SAT-323.

Index

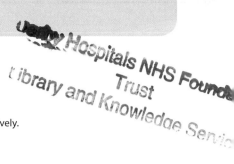

Note: Page numbers in **bold** or *italic* refer to tables or figures, respectively.